ADVANCE F

NEXT IN LINE

"A powerful analysis of the corporatization of medicine that could serve as the impetus for countering the forces destroying the rapport necessary for caregiver-patient relationships. The book elucidates how we got here and where we need to go."—**Henry Pohl, MD, Vice Dean for Academic Administration, Albany Medical College**

"If you believe that the physician-patient relationship is important–and especially if you do not believe this–then you should read this book. Timothy Hoff has drawn on his many years of study of physicians to write a passionate, cogent, compelling account–often in patients' and physicians' own words–of the forces that are threatening this relationship and of actions that could be taken to give physicians and patients a chance to make it stronger."—**Lawrence Casalino, MD, PhD, Professor of Healthcare Policy and Research, Weill Cornell Medical College**

"Picking up where he left off with his first book, *Practice under Pressure*, Prof. Hoff presents a compelling and extensively researched examination of the degradation of the physician-patient relationship as a result of the multiple forces rocking modern health care. Drawing upon his research and supplemented by interviews with primary care physicians, Hoff's timely analysis is especially relevant as organized medicine copes with widespread burnout of physicians and dissatisfaction of their patients. A cautionary work, this book should be required reading for physicians and policy makers alike who care about preserving the soul of medicine."—**Ephraim Back, MD, Clinical Professor, Albany Medical College**

"*Next in Line* is an insightful yet very objective assessment of the evolution of the doctor-patient relationship in the 21st century. Prof. Hoff, with his rational skepticism about the broken American health care system, listens to the voices of real patients and their doctors and leaves us with a prescription for fine tuning the dyadic doctor-patient relationship. *Next in Line* should be required reading for all from insurers to administrators and especially to physicians. Prof. Hoff's message comes through loud and clear—have faith in the art of medicine and keep the trust, listening, compassion, empathy, and mutual respect in the doctor-patient relationship."—**Denis Chagnon, MD, Past President, New York State Academy of Family Physicians**

"Timothy Hoff has written another excellent monograph on physicians. This book decries the burden to document quality imposed on our doctors by payers and policy-makers without regard for the damage done to the patient-physician relationship and critiques the emphasis on 'retail solutions' that shifts attention away from this relationship. More broadly, Prof. Hoff questions the general direction the health care system is taking, described by industry analysts as a transformation to 'value'. His critical analysis is on target. More people should be questioning this transformation, what value is being generated, and who benefits from it."—**Lawton Burns, PhD, Professor of Healthcare Management, University of Pennsylvania**

"Incisive analysis of what we need to preserve in the new world of team-based, performance-based health care delivery."—**Stephen Shortell, PhD, Professor of Organizational Behavior, University of California, Berkeley**

NEXT IN LINE

NEXT IN LINE

Lowered Care Expectations in the Age
of Retail- and Value-Based Health

Timothy J. Hoff, PhD

PROFESSOR OF MANAGEMENT, HEALTHCARE SYSTEMS,
AND HEALTH POLICY
D'AMORE-MCKIM SCHOOL OF BUSINESS
SCHOOL OF PUBLIC POLICY AND URBAN AFFAIRS
NORTHEASTERN UNIVERSITY
VISITING ASSOCIATE FELLOW
OXFORD UNIVERSITY

OXFORD
UNIVERSITY PRESS

OXFORD
UNIVERSITY PRESS

Oxford University Press is a department of the University of Oxford. It furthers
the University's objective of excellence in research, scholarship, and education
by publishing worldwide. Oxford is a registered trade mark of Oxford University
Press in the UK and certain other countries.

Published in the United States of America by Oxford University Press
198 Madison Avenue, New York, NY 10016, United States of America.

© Oxford University Press 2018

Library of Congress Cataloging-in-Publication Data
Names: Hoff, Timothy, 1965– author.
Title: Next in line : lowered care expectations in the age of retail- and
value-based health / Timothy J. Hoff.
Description: Oxford ; New York : Oxford University Press, [2018] |
Includes bibliographical references and index.
Identifiers: LCCN 2017012755 (print) | LCCN 2017014413 (ebook) |
ISBN 9780190626358 (updf) | ISBN 9780190626365 (epub) |
ISBN 9780190626341 (pbk. : alk. paper)
Subjects: | MESH: Primary Health Care | Physician-Patient Relations |
Quality of Health Care | Patient Satisfaction | Health Care Sector—trends | United States
Classification: LCC RA427.8 (ebook) | LCC RA427.8 (print) | NLM W 84.6 AA1 |
DDC 362.1—dc23
LC record available at https://lccn.loc.gov/2017012755

1 3 5 7 9 8 6 4 2
Printed by Webcom Inc., Canada

For Sharon and Kieran and My Mom and Dad

CONTENTS

CONTENTS

PREFACE

The doctor-patient relationship and the future of relational health care generally are not topics that have gotten the attention they deserve. One of my hopes is that this small contribution to informing these topics can encourage others to examine them in different ways. We talk so much about how important and sacrosanct the doctor-patient relationship is as a core feature of health delivery. Yet policy makers, industry executives, physicians, and patients seem to let it pass by them untouched. There is so much change occurring in health systems now around the world, so much of it unquestioned, that as patients *and* consumers we must get more interested. That interest should start with assessing our own ability to connect with doctors in a manner good for our health, and good for our overall feeling of well-being in both body and mind. We can hope we get the delivery system all of us deserve in the very near future, instead of the one others with profit-oriented reasons think we want or need. But to move there, the role of doctors as relational caregivers, and the role of this relational care in our lives, requires extended debate.

My chief motivation for conducting this study and turning it into a book is the growing concern I have as both a patient and health care scholar of where the U.S. health care delivery system is headed. By "headed" I mean more narrowly the direction our system is taking with respect to how to improve care quality and the "patient experience"; how to define notions of "value" within the system; how to conceptualize, manage, and evaluate medical work; the role of doctors and more general relationships in our care; and the increased power health care organizations are assuming over how care delivery is structured and reimbursed. In particular, I am concerned about how the traditional bedrock of this system, the doctor-patient relationship, is being affected by rapid change.

As described herein, things are moving quickly in health care. Whether it will be the Affordable Care Act or something else moving forward, one fact remains: the place of physicians in our health care lives and our ability to interact meaningfully with them is undergoing profound change. We see less of the doctor now when we access the health care system, presented instead with intermediaries of many different kinds, including technological interfaces, other personnel, and the larger organizations that house them both. Ongoing interactions with the same doctors over years are being replaced with more convenient but scattershot touch points with random doctors. These trends are accelerating. This is true especially in primary care. Of course, change is needed and good in any service industry like health care that for too long stayed mired in unproven tradition, costly and lower quality care, paternalism towards its customers, and too much physician control. But knowing that one situation must improve does not mean we shouldn't question what comes along to replace it, or that what arrives in its place is necessarily better because it is sold by a variety of self-interested stakeholders as the antidote to the less than perfect thing that came before it.

Today in health care we are "innovating" in many ways but questioning fewer of these innovations, even though much of what we are trying has little systematic empirical proof behind it. Most of the grand ideas seem to underperform and disappoint on a regular basis. In the past several years, we have had a major piece of legislation, the Affordable Care Act (ACA) that drove many of these changes. It has done some very good things in expanding health insurance, but has paid less attention to reforming the supply side of health care delivery. Thus, we see innovations such as patient-centered medical homes, accountable care organizations, value-based purchasing, team care, population health management, electronic health records, personalized health care—all of which are receiving much hype, policy attention, and resource infusion. Yet, at best they currently rest on a small and scattered body of weaker evidence, which does not indicate that they work reliably in achieving the kind of lofty goals set out for them in advance to gain support. The potential demise of the ACA may bring with it more unproven interventions for the system.

We talk knowingly about "how bad" the delivery system was when it was all about doctors or hospitals and their singular power. But now the technocrats, politicians, consultants, so-called experts, and industry executives support one idea after another with less regard for its proper design, implementation, or evaluation. Large employers, accrediting bodies like the National Committee for Quality Assurance, and insurance plans like Medicare throw their weight around dictating what health care quality should look like, drowning out physician and patient voices in the process. "Efficiency" becomes a treasured buzzword and goal, as if patient care could be work-flowed as easily as what occurs inside an Amazon fulfillment center. This produces a health care marketplace that comes across as increasingly impersonal and transactional; coldly calculating and corporate in its strategizing; and relying on half-baked policies and delivery "reforms" that lack a true appreciation for the deep complexity of health care work, as well as for what patients and doctors truly want to get out of experiencing that work.

Add to this a current state where patients are bewildered and dissatisfied about many aspects of the system they encounter; many health care professionals are unhappy and burned out in their jobs; health care costs remain high; and massive investment in a high-tech quality management infrastructure has fallen short in producing better or cheaper care. At the ground level, health care now seems to reproduce sub-par experiences for patients most of the time, as if this is the normal state of things. Maybe this is too strong or a somewhat biased critique. But it is the informed perspective of someone who has worked in the industry, studied it for over 20 years, and been a patient all his life.

In my 2010 book on primary care physicians, I sought to capture a part of the delivery system long neglected and under assault through the eyes of the professionals doing the work. I took an anthropological snapshot of a group of doctors that in 10 years will simply not do the same work, have the same roles, nor look the same way here in the United States. In fact, a lot of things already have changed since that book. The primary care system is morphing into something less personal and more transactional quicker than I thought. In that book, I illuminated how these physicians enacted their workdays and the ways in which that enactment was linked to changes in their values and belief systems regarding their careers, jobs, patients, and everyday work context. That book hinted at meaningful change in how doctors related to their patients. It and other related research prompted me to examine in greater depth this central facet of all physician work and legitimacy—the *relationship with patients*—that for decades has been held up as a sacrosanct and vital component of our system. The heart beating at the center of the health care delivery body, giving life and form to it.

Over the past several years, I have thought more about the doctor-patient relationship while witnessing this acceleration of "innovation" occurring in the industry, much of it arguably focused on saving or making stakeholders other than physicians and patients money; increasing transactional speed in health care to deal with rising patient demand; and pushing the principles of modern scientific management into as many aspects of the health care "production process" as possible. I constantly read about Silicon Valley entrepreneurs dabbling in health care "disruption," creating suspect products for people that are devoid of human contact and feel, but that sound cool and trendy. In my opinion, little policy or management attention has been given to maintaining or strengthening the doctor-patient relationship, or raising our expectations as patients for something warmer and more human. In fact, the construct of relationship often seems treated as an afterthought by everyone when discussing various reforms in the system. I worry about the view among some, particularly corporate interests and individual entrepreneurs with no previous health care interest or presence, to see health care as the next source of a major retail marketplace in our economy, that is, an array of as yet undefined yet potentially lucrative buying and selling opportunities, waiting for the right mix of resources, new thinking, and proper scale to occur. We should question that desire, and whether or not it is appropriate for health care. In my opinion, it is not.

The doctor-patient relationship as a construct has been largely ignored as a focus of empiricism, remaining more of an ideal-typical fantasy held in the hearts and minds of doctors and, perhaps, their patients.

This reality also has not played in its favor. It often is portrayed as a noble ideal rather than a practical necessity. As a result of the field's scholarly ambivalence about studying the concept in its totality, rather than its constituent parts, it has become easier to offer up solutions to system woes that neither acknowledge nor take advantage of the importance of this *social asset* in forging a better, *more humane* health care system. For example, so much of what the industry is now trying seems to consider the physician almost as an afterthought, a high-priced piece of labor requiring reeducation about how to perform their work in the correct (read: most efficient) manner. Patients have even less voice at the present time in terms of how the system should be structured to serve them, or to what extent they want physicians in their health care lives. This is disturbing for an industry that delivers the most personal of services to its clientele. It makes no sense.

In this light, it is useful to give the doctor-patient relationship and the evolving expectations of both these stakeholders additional scholarly treatment and apply what we learn to the practical realities of the present and future health care system. In this book, I provide a larger contextual analysis of what is happening to health care delivery in the United States, introduce the potential for "value-based" care, retail approaches, and "patient-as-consumer" thinking to take hold in a major way, and then weave in the voices of doctors and patients to help describe and assess their relational experiences, as well as their views on why such experiences are the norm. Variants of these system changes are also beginning to affect other international health systems such as in the United Kingdom and Canada, making the book broadly pertinent to a non-U.S. reading audience.

I intended this book to employ a "micro-level" analysis and then embed it within a "macro-level" contextual understanding of the various forces impinging on U.S. health care delivery at the present time. I thought this would be useful for better understanding why the doctor-patient relationship and our expectations regarding relational care are evolving in the manner discussed. The voices of doctors and patients speak to the future potential of relational care and a doctor-patient dyad that can engage in it. This book is focused on the primary care delivery system. But in reality that is pretty much where the notion of a strong dyadic relationship between doctor and patient can and should reach its highest potential. That said, its findings and lessons are relevant across all types of medical work.

Admittedly, this study is an incomplete treatment of a complex phenomenon. But it is a meaningful read for those interested in learning more about the most fundamental and traditionally important component of our health care delivery system, and its struggle for survival in a hostile environment. The implicit position taken from the outset is that this relationship has continued meaning and value for doctors, patients, health care quality and efficiency, and for increasing the moral and ethical integrity of our health care system. It is a vital thing to maintain and grow if our health care system is to be fairer, patient-centered, and more effective for each of us. But it may be on the verge of extinction. For those who may feel that focusing on the doctor-patient relationship is "old-fashioned" or "impractical" in a system embracing powerful information technology and analytics, machine learning, rational economic thinking, and scalable corporate care delivery, it still is worth a look, because it does provide convincing logic for a deeper debate about the specific direction in which health care delivery should be going.

This book owes many debts to individuals. First, the doctors and patients whom I interviewed merit sincere thanks. All of them were open, honest, and never held back in providing a wealth of interesting insights and experiences. I have worked with, studied, and taught doctors for a long time. I have great respect for what they do and how they go about doing it. It is a difficult job, yet many do it with a level of enthusiasm and commitment that is impressive. Those individuals who provided me with the patient perspective were a pleasure to speak with, and were all very aware of what they liked and did not like about their relationships with doctors, and interactions with the health care delivery system generally. I wish the industry talked more with us patients, because it would learn an awful lot it doesn't know at present.

My editor at Oxford University Press, Chad Zimmerman, was very supportive in encouraging me to write the book I was interested in writing. Both he and his assistant Chloe Layman were incredibly helpful in leading the project to fruition. Some ideas in the book, especially the focus on retail and consumer thinking in health care, were pilot tested through talks given at Green-Templeton College, Oxford University, where I am a

Visiting Associate Fellow; and at Northeastern University, where I am a Professor in the D'Amore-McKim School of Business and the School of Public Policy and Urban Affairs. These talks gave me the chance to have others offer their thoughts on some preliminary findings and the validity of the contextual backdrop described herein.

Most importantly, I cannot thank my wife Sharon and son Kieran enough for their support, not only for this book but throughout each day of my life. Academic work of this type can be a lonely endeavor. But their daily company make me feel excited and empowered to engage in my research and write these kinds of things. Sharon is a thoughtful sounding board for all of my work, and has been for over two decades. Kieran is a happy-go-lucky nine-year-old who obviously would always rather throw a football or shoot some hoops with me than talk about my work, and when he does want to read something the topic of our health care system is admittedly not in the forefront of his mind. Nevertheless, he gave me some good opinions on what I was doing, including asking me several times and quite pointedly, "Why are you doing this?" A more important question cannot be found when one is writing a book. I could not do stuff like this without their help. Finally, and as always, my parents deserve all the thanks in the world for helping to place me in a position to fulfill my career aspirations as a health care scholar, through their support, sacrifice, and investment in my preparation.

Chapter 1

Doctor-Patient Relationships and Our Expectations

I have to admit, my own interactions, and those of family members and friends with the primary care system over the past several years have been nothing to write home about. An increasingly interpersonally sterile, time-limited, low-expectation affair. It is full of reams of paper and e-mail notifications in the form of test results, physician instructions, and canned snippets about how to take care of myself, but short on any sort of relational warmth, genuine compassion, deep trust, or active listening—all things an effective doctor-patient relationship is supposed to be built upon. I rarely see my own primary care physician any more, and when I do, it does not feel very personable. In fact, it feels cold and distant.

In part, that's a key motivation for this book. The saying "write about what you know" holds here. In addition to my own local experiences, I see through my research and academic work what is happening to the U.S. primary care system, particularly in terms of the forces impinging on it; how it chooses to view and interact with patients; and how it treats its most important human capital, namely, physicians. It makes me uneasy. It should make all of us uneasy. Uneasy because the players increasingly driving innovation are outsiders, often companies and people who perhaps have too much of an interest in profit and growth; or government agencies like the Centers for Medicare and Medicaid Services that work off of little hard evidence at the same time they try one magic bullet after another for solving what ails our health system. All the while, the medical profession seems to sit on the sidelines, and although it has an interest in profit and growth, its individual members also assume a moral obligation to think bigger and act in our interests as patients.

Things are happening quickly to transform the entire primary care service delivery sector, and along with that the *doctor-patient relationship* in primary care, and no one is critiquing it much. But those involved feel it. In a recent survey of over 25,000 physicians nationwide, over half believed that the ongoing erosion of the doctor-patient relationship was a very important reason for their own perceived decline in the medical profession (Physicians Biannual Survey 2012). In a similar survey, almost 80 percent of the over 20,000 physicians surveyed stated that their relationship with patients was the most satisfying aspect of medical practice (Physicians Biannual Survey 2014). As a sociologist and student of the workplace, and someone who worked in the health care industry, I defer to what the workers think, not only because it makes sense in a service industry but also because of a wealth of academic research over the years that proves the accuracy of the worker view to how the real world operates. Many academics and practitioners celebrate all the innovation disrupting the business of primary care, but fewer of us understand for sure what positive or negative effects such innovation may bring to the transformation of medicine as a caring, human-to-human profession.

Of all the various branches of medicine, primary care is the proverbial canary in the coal mine for what is coming to the rest of health care over the next couple of decades (Hoff 2010a; 2013a). The big picture of health care transformation in the United States involves the hand of larger corporate entities bringing their ideology and business models to redesigning health care delivery. Part of that transformation involves the injection of retail philosophies into primary care; philosophies that will hasten a shift away from having patients interact primarily with their doctors, instead giving their loyalties over to a variety of targets such as doctors, non-physician providers, semiskilled health personnel such as medical assistants and, perhaps most importantly, the larger health care organization and system upon which we all increasingly rely to access care (Lazerow 2014).

These new relationships will be established with *systems* rather than with *individuals*, potentially de-emphasizing interpersonal attributes such as trust, communication, and empathy, and with the physician playing a less exclusive role in each health care transaction. These system relationships depend more on how we experience and perceive *the brand* or reputation of institutions employing an army of technological gadgets and salaried workers to provide us with "value" across an array of products and services (Estupinan, Kaura & Fengler 2014). They do not depend so much on ongoing social interaction with the same group of health care professionals or any one doctor but rather on the experiences associated with repeat purchases and transactional stability in the exchanges we have with the organization. In short, the future U.S. health care system, particularly in primary care, increasingly may grow to feel more like other consumer experiences we have in our lives, such as being an Amazon, Netflix, or Marriott customer.

GIVING TESTIMONY AROUND THE DOCTOR-PATIENT EXPERIENCE

A couple of years ago, when I ruptured my quadriceps tendon, I didn't think to touch base with my primary care physician (PCP) for advice or assessment. My insurance didn't require me to, and I didn't see the value in it, particularly because I had to make a time-limited set of decisions. One reason was that I was moving to a different town and wanted to get surgery there anyway. That's the easy answer. But it was more than that. Even if I had not been moving, I would not have called my existing PCP, because I believed he could do little for me. I also did not feel close to him, although he had been my "regular" PCP for over five years.

I felt this way partially because I hadn't seen him much, but then again I felt this was not my fault. He seemed increasingly walled off in his practice behind modern health workflow innovations such as nurse practitioners and team-based care delivery. Of course, my particular injury was beyond his pay grade to fix anyway. I knew from reading on the Internet that it would require surgery. But it was really more about my impression of inaccessibility. Had I called his office, my past experiences told me that it would have been impossible to get in to see him during those first crucial days. I also knew that I didn't have the kind of rapport or emotional bond with him that I imagined I wanted. Part of that was simply the lack of direct contact with him. I saw him generally once a year for a physical, where I got asked the rote questions and given the standard lab tests insurers and evidence-based care guidelines required to gauge my general health in the early 21st century, and that was about it. Maybe I was asked a couple of unique questions about myself at these annual exams, but they often seemed forced or orchestrated, and so I tended never to open up to him. Maybe that wasn't his fault. But I still blamed him for it.

That said, I continued to hope, and to convince myself that I needed a good, consistent relationship with a single primary care physician; a relationship in which I actually could get to know the physician and they could get to know me as a person. With that in mind, awhile back, I awoke on a brutally cold winter morning resolved to address the upper-respiratory problem that had been making me feel lousy for going on a four-week period. Now living outside of Boston, I picked up the phone and made the call to my new regular primary care physician (PCP), the one with whom I had had to wait four months to get a new patient appointment. Of course, I could have decided that morning to visit my local retail clinic or urgent care center. There's an increasing number of those options where I live. But I felt that my PCP was the best option to diagnose and treat something I had now had for going on a month.

Part of me felt something more serious could be wrong. Don't we all think that at times, even if it's irrational? I wanted the person I saw as my personal physician expert, even if I did not know her well yet, to help assure me that everything was fine. For some reason I felt that she could make me understand what, if anything was wrong with me, and that seeing her would have added value for the assessment of my illness. In hindsight, though, what I thought I wanted got the better of me once again. First, I was delusional in my thinking that someone I had seen only a few times over a two-year period was really my dedicated health coach and advisor— which by the way is a role primary care physicians are expected to play in new models of care such as the patient-centered medical home—or knew me better than anyone else did in the health care system.

I probably should have gotten into my car and gone to one of those other places, where convenience and timely access would have been better. At least there would have been no expectation on my part of getting something I felt I deserved, or chasing something that for me did not exist in reality. Because the call to my primary care physician's office that day was, as I had feared, a 15-minute frustration fest that did not seem focused on enabling me to see *my doctor*. Instead, it came across as a pre-scripted attempt to guess my clinical situation up front, drop me into a preordained diagnostic category, and then funnel me into a scheduled slot of the office's choosing, not mine.

First, I got the cold, recorded voice that sent me through several button-pushes on the phone, ending with my leaving a voice mail with my doctor's assistant. A half hour later, called back at the beginning of what was a busy workday for me, I came into contact with a non-clinical assistant and was put through a highly standardized form of generic triage. The front-desk person with whom I was speaking, kind in demeanor but unable to offer specific advice of any kind given the person's non-clinical status, was allowed only to respond to every question or request with standard responses such as "Dr. X has no available appointments for the next two weeks, but we could fit you in with our nurse practitioner tomorrow," and "I can't give you any advice on your condition, but we can try and fit you in for an appointment with another provider in the next couple of days." This was the entire substance of our back and forth for those few minutes.

Already unable to communicate electronically with my physician in a timely fashion (i.e., getting an answer within a few hours, rather than in a day or days) despite their practice having an electronic medical record and a patient portal; and unable to see my personal physician today or tomorrow for a condition seemingly minor in the eyes of the screener but worrying me, I voiced my dissatisfaction and got off the phone. In the end, I didn't go anywhere. Instead, I lived with my symptoms for another week before they gradually began to ebb permanently. As another doctor had told me once before, 80 percent of what's wrong with patients gets better on its own with time. In this instance, my symptoms fell into that 80 percent. Lucky me.

But what if something more serious had been wrong? What if the symptoms I experienced for a month were proxies for a type of cancer, or some debilitating metabolic condition, or pneumonia? What if they were outgrowths of an underlying behavioral condition such as depression or too much stress in my life? What if something about how I was living my life at that particular moment was facilitating my getting sick, how would that have been unearthed and acted upon by the local urgent care center or retail clinic that didn't know me? Sure, these places somehow might have picked up these things. But likely not. Even if they had been noticed, these facilities would have directed me back to my primary care doctor, because that's what they do. They provide episodic, not continuous care.

Contrast my own experiences with those of a close family member, a recently diagnosed diabetic. The thing to remember about high-cost chronic diseases in the modern age of primary care is that if you are unfortunate enough to have such a disease, you may get much better attention from your primary care doctor and practice, at least temporarily, than if you presented as generally healthy, even if your body was brewing up some terrible affliction that remained hidden. But attention from your doctor in today's health system does not always translate into the opportunity to cultivate a deep, trusting, and empathetic relationship. Rather, with chronic disease you become part of a bigger "population," that is, a disease as well as an individual, and a series of "big data" metrics requiring ongoing monitoring and control. We give this reality an appealing name, *population health management*. Although it has achieved success in terms of assuring that diabetics, hypertensives, and other chronic disease groups get a certain level of appropriate, standardized care directed at them, it may be one of the more insidious ways in which the individual-level doctor-patient relationship in primary care is being undercut.

My family member was receiving largely the same type of non-physician centric primary care as I was, until she got type 2 diabetes. Discovering this disease moved her to the top of the PCP's interest list, at least initially. The first few months after being diagnosed, and with a Hemoglobin A1C well above the guideline-appropriate number of seven, which is the standard "quality outcome" in most insurers' performance management systems (National Institute of Diabetes and Digestive and Kidney Disorders 2014), she was able to make several in-person visits to her primary care doctor. In addition, the primary care office called her back and left messages for her in the electronic patient portal in a timely manner after she left questions or requests, and she had several long visits discussing her diabetes and overall lifestyle situation with the doctor. However, once her blood sugar was under control, that is, after her A1C number fell under the magic seven benchmark, this attention waned. The next time she had to go into the practice for another complaint, she was not able to see her own personal physician. Instead, she once again (as happened before her diabetes diagnosis) got plugged into a visit with the physician assistant. She still gets to see her primary care doctor periodically, but those sporadic visits are built entirely around checking her diabetes numbers, or having her annual physical.

THE NEW NORMAL OF PRIMARY CARE

Running a primary care practice today means being efficient and streamlining the delivery of services in whatever ways possible. For example, patients are sorted into different groups of care needs, both ahead of time using data and when they contact their doctor's office directly. The latter is called "triage" and often is done over the phone and increasingly performed by a lower-level, non-physician staff person. In fewer instances, primary care physicians make these initial up-front decisions about what to do with a patient concern, turning responsibility over to standardized care pathways and written policies they invent to manage workload. Private insurers and government payers like Medicare influence these pathways and policies through their rules and payment policies. For most primary care doctor's offices, where reimbursements sometimes barely cover costs and profit margins may be razor-thin, keeping individuals away from a face-to-face visit with the doctor is often an implicit goal. In the modern primary care system, the doctor is the high-cost labor input in a production process that remains underfunded and overwhelmed by demand. Increasingly, insurers question the value of patients needing to see their doctor for all but the most important clinical situations, as they (the insurers) define those.

Thus, the triage process, so much a part of our interactions with the health care system, often involves connecting patients with their doctor only in special circumstances, namely, those (a) that maximize the reimbursement gained from using more complex billing codes (a rarity these days in primary care given that most office visit reimbursement is fixed by a limited set of codes); (b) where chronic diseases must be managed carefully so that physicians can report the right kinds of performance metrics to insurers to get additional reimbursement or not be financially penalized; or (c) those where patients require annual physical exams that still produce good reimbursement, and allow the doctor to check up on sicker patients who impact the office performance metrics disproportionately. For all other patient situations, the norm is deflection and getting plugged into lower-cost options, even if that means implicitly convincing many patients to stay home and wait to see how their illness progresses.

We call most primary care practices "patient-centered medical homes" now, as if that moniker denotes an innovative, warm, and trusting place where we have satisfying access to our doctors when we think we need it (Hoff 2013b). I have heard from many primary care physicians and their staff members in my own research that being labeled a medical home involves dressing up a practice to show an accrediting agency that you have checked the correct boxes on a several-page checklist regarding which work processes or policies are in place in the practice (Hoff 2010b; 2013b). For instance, checking the box that says you have a written patient access policy doesn't prove patients can actually access *their own doctor* in a timely way. The medical practice must *assign* everyone a personal physician for their care, as required by another checkbox, but it doesn't have to prove to the outside world that people are allowed to see that personal physician when they want.

Within this new world of primary care, where offices are called inviting names like "medical homes" at the same time that they seek to remove their patients' physicians from plain view, my experience on that winter day involved running into a staff person strategically placed to interfere with my desire to see my doctor. I encountered an office that showed a general disregard for trying to cultivate any sort of meaningful connection between me as a patient and my doctor. There was no other way for me to perceive it. No doubt driven by their own capacity limitations and financial imperatives, staff in that office likely would see their interaction with me on that day as very rational. Or, they simply wouldn't care about my perceptions, instead worried more about getting through the workday and getting the office buttoned down for the evening at a reasonable hour. Policy makers and industry executives also might think the same. As a patient, however, I came away thinking that the primary goal for that office, and by implication my personal physician, was to give everyone the same cheapened and impersonal level of service delivery, all presumably in the name of noble-sounding concepts like "timely access" (which I didn't get that day), "better care quality" (which I didn't get because I didn't gain access), and "efficiency" (which the office may have gained but which I as a patient couldn't care less about when I didn't feel well). These three system goals look great on paper but are lousy when pursued on an everyday basis in American health care. Ironically, the entire experience left me in a situation where I remained sick, chose not to seek care, and came away with even less confidence, trust, and feeling of closeness to *my doctor* than ever.

Maybe I was part of the problem, too. As I alluded to earlier, did I expect too much as a patient? Did I imagine a fantasy-world for myself where I could have a physician who knew me, knew my family (it is called family medicine, isn't it?), and whom I trusted to give me clinical (and perhaps life) advice tailored to my needs, life circumstances, personality, and motivation? Convenience; timely access to my doctor, rather than well-intended office staff who were not in a position to make informed decisions about my care; and a doctor who wanted to and could spend time with me—was this an unrealistic vision? I had begun to think so, because for a few years now, the traditional primary care physician's office was failing on all these fronts in significant ways. So another part of me has begun to feel as though it is time to try other ways of doing primary care that perhaps do not involve a personal physician or even a doctor's office at the heart of it. Something new and different perhaps.

But that's the potential trap—new and different likely will not ever get me back to the strong personal desire I have for a deeper, ongoing relationship with a single doctor. Because while policy makers and self-interested stakeholders like industry executives, physician associations, think tanks, and foundations embrace the retail concept and other ideas out there such as the patient-centered medical home or team-based care, they are casting a blind eye to how these ideas further undermine the *relational* aspects of care, particularly those aspects that involve social interaction between individual patients and their doctors. Most of the time, what I've learned is that these kinds of stakeholders don't want to know what they don't know, because to know more reveals head-hurting complexity in areas they are trying to simplify for the sake of solving problems quickly.

In this way, the preoccupation in promoting various primary care innovations, for example, tends to focus on low-hanging fruit such as basic quality of care and patient satisfaction indicators, reducing emergency department use and unnecessary hospital admissions, and the dollar costs of providing a given service. A quick glance through the literature evaluating some of these innovations proves this point (Alexander and Bae 2012; Ashwood et al. 2016; Grumbach and Bodenheimer 2004; Hoff, Weller, and DePuccio 2012; Jacoby et al. 2011). On the other hand, you will find few studies assessing in-depth how such innovations affect the substantive aspects of the doctor-patient *relationship*, namely, features such as trust, empathy, communication, listening, emotional bonds, or the depth of knowledge on the physician's part of a patient's life situation and psychological makeup.

The new normal of primary care involves a lot of disruptive innovation. The general idea behind disruptive innovation is to do something more cheaply for consumers that the existing marketplace is ignoring, or doesn't do very well but is important to the consumer. In health care, care delivery disruptions include non-physician led retail clinics, urgent care centers, web applications that promote access to care such as ZocDoc and Doctor on Demand, wearable health technology like FitBits, electronic health records, and population health management strategies that use big data to segment and identify patients in need. Many of these innovations de-emphasize a stable and ongoing doctor-patient relationship that contains highly relational features. They simply do not incorporate such a concept into their business models or underlying philosophy of how to meet patient needs and expectations.

Instead, the things of value become more transactional and less relational; for example, quick and convenient access to service, regardless of who is doing the responding and resolving, or even if it has a high likelihood of preventing a second patient interaction with the delivery system, and consistent service delivery that provides a similar level of transactional satisfaction to the patient each time. The practical and even moral justifications supporting the value of strong interpersonal relationships in health care between individual doctors and their patients give way to the strategic logic for making health care delivery more *available* (which increases the revenue that can be extracted from patients in a given time period) and the patient *transaction* more reliable in terms of speed and execution (which enhances the capacity for a health care organization or system to absorb demand, control its patients' service use more tightly, and gain greater market share in the process). Through this lens, it makes sense to find ways to get the physician out of the care delivery workflow, if only to lower per unit costs of the transaction itself.

In fairness to these innovations, they simply take advantage of the reality that few seem to care much right now about promoting strong doctor-patient relationships in medicine, because no one is implementing the extended structural, financial, and cultural changes within the system that would support them. And high costs and patient access remain front-and-center issues, so anything that promises cheaper or timelier care delivery is embraced. In addition, at a macro level, quality-of-care problems festered for too long, opening the door to introducing new approaches. In this way, electronic health records, the use of team care, the use of clinical guidelines and standardized performance metrics, and population-based health management all have their place in so far as they can improve quality in some meaningful way.

Another part of the narrative supporting a turn away from maintaining a strong doctor-patient relationship at the heart of health care delivery toward pursuing other system goals is that for too long the U.S. health care system was a "Wild West" full of a fair portion of cowboy doctors who used the term "doctor-patient relationship" as a shield to deflect those outside interests seeking to make medical work more transparent and doctors more accountable. These doctors liked to run their offices the way they wanted, didn't do things in a particularly cost-effective way, eschewed transparency in how they provided care, didn't like to follow guidelines and provide standardized care where it made sense to do so, treated patients too paternalistically, and were preoccupied with compensation. They also embraced a "do more, get more" payment philosophy through fee-for-service medicine, and did not always put their patients' interests first.

Some of this narrative is true. But what it conveniently leaves out is that other stakeholders—government, third-party payers, employers, foundations, think tanks, corporations, and entrepreneurs—now seek greater influence in the system for their own self-interested reasons, which include control over how health care dollars are spent, greater market share and brand loyalty, and the desire to push specific ideologies on the health care public, for the purpose of advancing self-interested causes. This reality is accompanied by a collective desperation on the part of primary care physicians to hold onto their legitimacy at all costs, resulting in short-term strategic decisions (e.g., leaving hospital care altogether) that may enhance the financials of their business temporarily but come at the expense of the relationships they have with their patients, as well as their credibility and perceived value to the public (see Hoff 2010b).

It is within this context of needing to solve real problems, while embracing half-truths and allowing untested innovations to enter the health care market quickly that a lot of half-baked policy ideas have gained traction in primary care. The past two decades of underperforming but boldly promised ideas like managed care, capitation, pay-for-performance, medical homes, team-based care, and electronic medical records bear witness to that reality. Notice in this discussion I have not identified what individual patients say they want or do not want as a key driver of innovation at the present time. Their direct voice is still only tangential to the main conversation occurring, despite industry rhetoric around the importance of consumer engagement (Estupinan, Kaura & Fengler 2014), and payers such as Medicare assigning a dollar value to "patient experience" within their value-based reimbursement models (Centers for Medicare and Medicaid Services 2016b).

This book seeks out the voices of primary care physicians and their patients to examine the current state of the doctor-patient relationship in health care, in light of the changes occurring around it. What are we losing and what have we already lost? What is it about relational care that makes a difference, and does it really make a difference? Are my own set of experiences described earlier typical or exceptional? Is it more complicated or perhaps simpler than how I am framing it here? Do doctors and patients want the same things? What motivates people to have a certain kind of doctor-patient relationship, that is, the kind that fulfills both stakeholders who are a part of it? What will this relationship look like in the future? These are some of the questions explored in the remaining chapters. First, however, we need to know more about how the doctor-patient relationship has been conceptualized and in what ways it is seen as possessing value for those involved in it, as well as the health care system as a whole.

ROMANTIC YET REAL NOTIONS OF THE DOCTOR-PATIENT RELATIONSHIP IN PRIMARY CARE

Most physicians believe that their relationships with patients are the most satisfying aspects of their medical practice, so it matters to them (The Physicians Foundation 2014). But what is that relationship anyway? First, it's important to recognize that any relationship is a vague construct to specify. Relationships are hard to quantify, multidimensional in substance, consisting of psychological and behavioral features, and require extended periods of time to cultivate and assess. They are fluid, not static, evolving over time in unpredictable ways shaped by their surrounding contexts. This is especially true of *interpersonal* relationships, that is, the kind that exist between people rather than between people and organizations, for example.

Because they bear these qualities, interpersonal relationships do not lend themselves easily to systematic assessment or clear operational definitions. It may also be hard to ascribe clear value to them in the sense of knowing precisely how they impact different outcomes for the individuals involved. In a U.S. health care system that currently is both metric and standardization obsessed, this means that interpersonal relationships may go largely unnoticed. Certainly, there is little focus on the doctor-patient relationship within policy or management debates about which specific health care innovations to bring to market, which problems in the everyday clinical setting are most profound, and the best ways in which we should spend limited dollars for care delivery. Rather, the emphasis in these debates is on lowering the costs of care, streamlining how care is delivered, and actually removing the physician from select patient care work to achieve both of these goals.

Within the current context of neglect the relational features of patient care are oversimplified and made to seem easily preserved. Their current measurement within the industry shows this plainly. For example, there are standardized assessments, the most notable of which is the Consumer Assessment of Healthcare Providers and Systems (CAHPS) that assess things like how well you think your doctor communicated with or explained things to you at a particular visit. Many in the health care industry defend these types of static, incomplete measures, given that they are better than nothing, and despite the reality that they do not tap into the complex aspects of an ongoing doctor-patient *relationship* that should involve regular direct interaction. CAHPS asks each patient the same generic questions, and seek brief comment on a single encounter or short time frame with a provider who may or may not be the patient's regular physician (Centers for Medicare and Medicaid 2016a). It assesses elements of the health care *transaction*.

More recently, there is also increasing (though still not even close to widespread) use of social media platforms such as *Yelp!* that let patients provide brief reviews of their care experiences in hospitals and with specific doctors (Ranard et al. 2016). Overall, the measurement focus on the patient experience remains primitive at best. It does not help us better understand what particular aspects of a doctor-patient *relationship* are most valued by participants, nor does it serve as a means to intervene to maintain or cultivate relational care elements within medical offices. Instead, most care providers have been socialized by insurers and the government to use the results as a form of report card for which they can seek additional reimbursement for their services (Centers for Medicare and Medicaid Services 2016a).

The doctor-patient relationship has been written about in the medical literature frequently over the past 75 years. By and large, it has been romanticized by writers, mostly physicians, in ways that emphasize its healing aspects for the patient and cathartic value for the physician. This literature has highlighted in depth how the interpersonal features associated with good relational care between doctor and patient produce a range of important outcomes (see Hoff and Collinson 2016). Consider these various snippets from published literature on the topic:

> *The personal aspect of the doctor-patient relationship deals with the illness experience and the context of the patient's life. In effect, patients are the subjective experts on their illness experience, but may not know*

*how best to communicate this experience to the physician. As this rela-
tionship deals with the subjective experiences of both patient and physician, physicians have to rely exclusively upon their interpersonal skills to
assess the illness experience, but, for optimal treatment, physician and
patient must reach a common understanding about the illness experience. (Botelho 1992: 212)*

*The perception of the physician by most patients in the past and largely
still existent, despite adverse publicity on the deteriorating role of the
physician, is that the physician is a healer, often a friend, a confidant and
a trusted clinical advisor. This last role is crucial and indicates that the
physician will hold the patient's illness of first concern, not the concerns
of society or of the health care system itself. (Turino 1986: 1015)*

*The doctor/patient relationship is based on the part of the doctor on
expertise, authority and humanity and on the part of the patient on
expectation and trust. The doctor has the greater responsibility for its
development; it should remain under his or her control but he or she
must remember that it is a partnership and be receptive to the patient's
input. The professional contribution will depend on personality, knowledge of patients' psychology and behaviour, skills and attitudes. The
doctor's personality should reflect an interest in people tempered with
compassion, warmth and humility, and his or her knowledge of patients
should extend to their beliefs in health, their expectations, their preferences, their desire for independence, their trust, shame, fears and guilt.
Of all the skills required, by far the most important is the ability to communicate, to be able to talk, listen, observe, and to develop understanding
and insight. (King 1987: 591)*

*In general practice, reassurance forms a large part of the treatment. In
this the doctor's own personality means much. If he can instill confidence
into a patient, the latter will believe him when told that there is no cause
for worry. (Shorten 1966: 33)*

*The relation between a physician and his patient is one which necessarily
requires that the patient make a full and frank disclosure to his physician of intimate, personal and private information in order that the latter can make an informed diagnosis and render proper treatment. The*

relationship, therefore, is one of trust and confidence and requires the physician to exercise the utmost good faith and fair dealing in his relations with his patient. (Challener 1949: 624)

What is clear from reading this literature is that the doctor-patient relationship represents to many, especially physicians, a social contract of the highest order between expert professional and vulnerable individual—a social contract gaining legitimacy from the patient entrusting certain roles to physicians (e.g., knowledge broker, listener, healer, confidante, advisor) in return for physicians committing themselves to the patient's interests and taking keen interest in maximizing their potential to lead healthy lives. Literature on the doctor-patient relationship emphasizes features such as trust, information, listening, empathy, communication, compassion, autonomy, respect, and confidentiality as integral to a mutually rewarding relationship (Hoff and Collinson 2016; Keating et al. 2002). It also emphasizes the social and psychological aspects that go into the creation and maintenance of that relationship.

Of all features, *trust* is perhaps most central to the doctor-patient relationship. Trust is generally defined as one party's willingness to be vulnerable to another's behavior with the expectation that the former will benefit from that behavior (Mayer, Davis, and Schoorman 1995). At the core of trust are two key aspects: (a) vulnerability (Hall et al. 2001) and (b) expectation (Morgan and Hunt 1999). Hall and colleagues (2001) note the importance of trust in the doctor-patient relationship:

Intrinsically, it is the core, defining characteristic that gives the doctor-patient relationship meaning, importance, and substance—the way love or friendship defines the quality of an intimate relationship. . . . trust is widely believed to be essential to effective therapeutic encounters (p. 613–614).

Trust is positively associated with patient engagement with their own health and care, as well as a greater likelihood of patients to remain with their physicians (Becker and Roblin 2008; Thom and Campbell 1997; Trachtenberg, Dugan, and Hall 2005). It looms large as a predictor of a more positive patient experience with serious diagnoses such as mental illness and cancer (Schroeder 2013). Trust is also an important intangible that allows patients to participate as coequals in the clinical encounter, and experience greater openness and honesty with their physicians. Patient trust in physicians increases adherence and compliance to treatment regimens (Hall et al. 2001; Thom and Campbell 1997). In addition, as Hall et al. (2001) note, trust in the doctor-patient relationship may mediate clinical outcomes by shaping the relative impact of various therapeutic interventions, for example, through its value in getting patients to believe in the treatment provided to them, even before tangible results are seen.

There are two main types of trust, calculative and relational. Relational trust is the trust spoken about in the literature as integral to an effective doctor-patient relationship. Relational trust is stronger, more interpersonal, and more organic in nature, built over time through positive, mutually reinforcing experiences individuals have with each other that build up repositories of goodwill, intimacy, and mutual respect. Given that it is experientially forged, relational trust depends greatly upon ongoing social interaction between doctor and patient. In one research study, such trust was enhanced through longer consultations between doctor and patient, as well as by the physician's own verbal behavior during the encounter (Fiscella et al. 2004).

Calculative trust is the kind of trust now underlying innovations in payment related to financially incentivizing doctors and their work, and which are called by names such as "pay-for-performance" or "value-based purchasing." Calculative trust is rooted in economic interactions between people and/or organizations that involve the exchange of goods for payment. A good could consist of enhanced performance on a given set of performance metrics, for example. Giving primary care physicians a financial bonus for making sure they test their diabetic patients' blood sugar every three months, or achieve an outcome of ensuring their diabetic patients as a group have average Hemoglobin A1C's under seven (the gold standard used) are examples of calculative trust in action. Insurers (and patients) can expect doctors to do the testing and proactively try to get everyone to below seven because there is a tangible reward if they do (or penalty if they don't), and if the reward is not there, some may not do it in a timely manner.

This trust is purely instrumental, that is, derived solely from the presence of the reward and people's expectations that physicians will comply with the requirements for reward. It is not rooted in ongoing social interaction or dependent upon other relational features, such as empathy or listening, being evident. It also is more inherently unstable than relational trust, given its Pavlovian nature and the lack of an interpersonal foundation around it that produces interactions between people that convey these other relational features. Through calculative trust, a doctor may get a group of diabetic patients to have all of their A1C levels taken within the required time period, but those patients may not motivate themselves to further action in improving their A1C level, or any other aspect of their overall health, in the absence of a deeper faith (verified through prior interactions) that their physician cares about them, wants to know them as a unique person, and is doing things specifically in their best interests (rather than in the insurers' best interests, for instance).

Relational trust depends on things like communication, compassion, empathy, and listening occurring between doctor and patient. These are interrelated features of the doctor-patient relationship that also are shown as beneficial for patients, in part because they help in the trust development process but also because they stand alone as positive predictors of better health outcomes. Take communication—why is doctor-patient communication so important? Kaplan et al. (1989) state:

> Beyond the obvious—the transfer of the information patients need to manager their disease effectively—the communication between physicians and patients can be a source of motivation, incentive, reassurance, and support as well as an opportunity for revision of expectations of both patient and physician. For many, if not most, patients the physician represents a formidable source of power and influence. As such, the physician may be in a unique position not only to influence the patient's technical care and to persuade the patient to follow the dictates of that care, but also to change patients' perceptions of their health status and beliefs about and self-confidence regarding their ability to influence their health status and to provide motivation and incentives for engaging in health promotion (S112).

In a review of various communication behaviors in health care delivery, Street et al. (2009) identified several studies that showed associations between physician-patient communication behaviors and outcomes such as lower blood pressure (Orth et al. 1987); decreased patient anxiety (Fogarty et al. 1999); and improved quality of life among cancer patients (Street and Voigt 1997). Kaplan et al. (1989) also found that effective physician-patient communication favorably impacted outcomes such as blood pressure, blood sugar levels in diabetics, and symptom experience with chemotherapy. The quality of doctor-patient communication also has been shown to improve information exchange and compliance in cancer care (Baile and Aaron 2005). Effective physician-patient communication positively impacts patients' emotional health, aids in symptom resolution and pain control, and impacts a variety of physiological measures (Beck, Daughtridge, and Sloane 2002; Stewart 1995). Still another review of over 500 separate patient visits found that communication consisting of physician reassurance of patient concerns was associated with better overall health (Fassaert et al. 2008).

As Stewart (1995) notes, the *quality* of doctor-patient communication matters. For example, Kaplan et al. (1989) found that communication involving higher levels of patient control, lower levels of physician control, greater involvement by the patient, and greater physician information sharing impacted select health outcomes more favorably than communication that did not possess these attributes. Some communication behaviors found particularly effective involve those that embody high degrees of compassion, question asking, and empathy toward patients. Empathy, defined as a psychological process involving the ability of one party to share feelings and experiences with another party, and having the latter be able to identify with those feelings and experiences, is linked to more effective diagnosis, better health outcomes, and an enhanced patient experience (Derksen, Bensing, and Lagro-Janssen 2013; Di Blasi et al., 2001; Hoff 2010b). Physicians who use their communication opportunities with patients to dialogue around the latter's concerns and expectations reduce patient anxiety as well as various symptoms (Stewart 1995).

Active listening, in which the physician takes in information from the patient in the course of a dialogue that helps to better understand the latter's needs and concerns, also is a key part of communication that improves outcomes (Baile and Aaron 2005). Patients prefer communication with their physicians that involves active listening (Van Berckelaer et al. 2012). Ong et al. (1995) identified the importance of communication that provided technical information between doctor and patient, that is, information directly impacting correct diagnosis and treatment. In addition, communication that conveys emotional support for patients is received better, and can decrease feelings of uncertainty, quell anxieties, and improve patient satisfaction (Simpson et al. 1991).

For the above reasons, Simpson et al. (1991) state that communication between doctor and patient cannot be delegated. It is interpersonal, and arguably best nurtured through interactions that are given adequate time, are mostly synchronous and face-to-face, and occur between the same individuals with some semblance of prior history. Communication involving empathy, emotional support, and active listening are most central to the physician's work, because it helps their ability to be perceived as the legitimate authority to diagnose and treat. This is an important point. It means that although patients today may increasingly encounter communication directly from health care organizations, or clinical teams made up of multiple non-physician personnel, it is still communication coming directly and firsthand from the physician that evidence shows and logic dictates is linked to a variety of positive outcomes, and to establishing the very trust between doctor and patient vital to the therapeutic endeavor.

In short, the *physician's* provision of emotional support through personal communication with patients matters. The *physician's* empathy and listening through personal communication with patients activates patients and helps them self-manage and comply. It is the *physician's* compassion and interest in the patient's concerns, conveyed through personal communication with patients that engenders patient trust in them. This makes sense, especially if we are comfortable with the notion that we still access medical care to gain input from the doctor, with everyone else in the system at best serving as conduits for that connection. In addition, and this has implications for the retail philosophy discussed in Chapter 3, each patient has to be understood in terms of the patient's unique context, since each may require a different communication or listening strategy tailored to the individual; and each has different needs for empathy, control, or involvement depending on his or her own circumstances (Mazzi et al. 2015).

Besides the conceptual logic and empirical proof, relational elements such as trust, respect, communication, listening, and empathy possess heavy doses of face validity when it comes to thinking about the roles they play in facilitating a variety of positive outcomes for both patients and doctors. In other words, although it is important to show that we can explain abstractly why certain interpersonal features of a doctor-patient relationship matter, or cite empirical facts that link them to specific patient benefits, common sense tells us that if they are important in other walks of life, then they should enhance our interactions with the trained professionals we seek out in health care, law, and other areas of our lives that involve personal vulnerability of some sort. Do family relationships work better, and yield greater rewards for all involved, when they are characterized by meaningful amounts of interpersonal trust, compassion, or empathy? Do we think that paying our siblings or children extra to behave in ways that we desire generates long-term trust with them, or produces long-term changes in other behaviors beyond the reach of that incentive? Does a higher-quality marriage on average result from effective communication, involving active listening, for example, between spouses? Do our jobs and work-related outputs, as well as our own feelings of satisfaction benefit from a social environment in which we and our coworkers, and our bosses, listen to one another, trust why certain decisions have to be made, and communicate regularly?

If we are honest, then the answers to these types of questions support the vital role these relational features play in our interactions with others. So, too, with physicians, because health care relationships are *healing relationships,* which means they serve an important purpose in our lives. Yet, as we will see, the doctor-patient relationship is not the only connection patients in our health system are encouraged to accept and participate in any more. Increasingly, patients are asked to engage with organizations, other types of health care workers who may be less skilled than physicians but are part of the *health care team,* and even larger systems whose brand names (e.g., Kaiser Permanente, Mayo, Brigham and Women's) are intended in part to convey features such as reliability, trust, and even compassion. The retail or consumer engagement movement in health care is predicated in part on transferring the notion of *relationship* from doctor-patient to patient-organization, and patient-brand, with the emphasis on creating a multifaceted buying experience with many different aspects of that single organization, and long-term allegiance to an impersonal symbol of general excellence (e.g., the name of the institution).

We must question this tectonic shift, and do it in the context of understanding what we may be losing or gaining with respect to the *doctor-patient relationship* and the relational care features associated with that relationship, which have been the foundation of our health care experience for decades. In the field of primary care particularly, there is a strong case to be made that the physician and patient must by necessity cultivate and maintain the relational features described above, for the benefit of both groups. Why? As patients, we are more prone than ever to disease and illness, to leading unhealthy lives in a complex society that demands much of each one of us and exposes us to many different forms of risk. We face a fragmented health care delivery system in which individual patients get turned into population segments of generically similar statistics, for purposes of providing cheaper standardized service delivery. We suffer greater stress and depression as human beings, and some compassionate entity in the health care system has to understand us as unique individuals, our life experiences, and our personalities, for these issues to get appropriately identified, managed, and resolved. In theory, it is still the primary care system that can tie it all together for us, and offer perhaps a place for singular, comprehensive attention to our needs.

Exploring whether and how the doctor-patient relationship in primary care matters, and whether that relationship is now based more in fantasy and wishful thinking than real experience, comprises the focus of this book. The voices of primary care physicians and patients tell us what this relationship means to them, why it's important, and how it is being impacted by changes in the health care system, paying special attention to certain system forces and how they breed fertile ground for growing the retail philosophy, with its attention to creating "consumers" out of patients. Before hearing these voices, however, we need to understand the current health care context better. The next two chapters analyze some of the more important changes in greater depth.

Chapter 2

The Forces Impacting
Doctor-Patient Relationships
and Our Expectations

No other part of the U.S. health care system is transforming more at present than primary care. This chapter describes and analyzes key environmental forces driving this transformation. These forces have implications for the doctor-patient relationship, and for the viability of preferred features in that relationship outlined in Chapter 1. Although primary care is affected most by these forces, they impact all parts of the health care delivery system. They are: (a) the establishment of a widespread "health care quality machine" that gives legitimacy to modern techniques of standardized quality measuring and reporting, spurring an emphasis on value-based reimbursement and creating "metric fever" in the industry; (b) large-scale efforts to integrate health care services and physicians into new, complex delivery structures such as Patient-Centered Medical Homes and Accountable Care Organizations, in theory to enhance the value of lower-cost services such as primary care but which also places more physicians at the mercy of the corporate organizations; and (c) patient access issues spurred by the Affordable Care Act's expansion of the insurance market, and exacerbated by long-standing primary care physician (PCP) supply problems, leading to further disruptive innovations such as retail clinics and the use of non-physician providers that downplay the physician role in care delivery.

The "Triple Aim" of lowered care costs, improved population health, and enhanced patient experiences, adopted by the industry as its bumper sticker slogan to make health care better gives these forces an additional aspect of importance (Institute for Healthcare Improvement 2016). The Triple Aim mantra helps to justify the multifaceted array of system imperatives that must now be addressed in the U.S. system. No longer is it appropriate to simply worry about quality but not costs, for example, or efficiency without a better patient experience. In theory, the Triple Aim has inherent appeal. Its system emphasis encourages pursuits such as population health management, organizational integration, care standardization, and disruptive innovation that lowers the costs of care. But it also de-emphasizes the potential worth of dyadic doctor-patient relationships. In its own concept design document, for example, the word "physician" never even appears, and the more vaguely understood term "provider" shows up only a couple of times (Institute for Healthcare Improvement 2016). Instead, the emphasis is on seeing individual patients as members of larger homogenous groups, and seeing doctors as part of health care teams. It does not speak to the need to preserve relational care between doctor and patient.

These forces redistribute power and influence within primary care in ways worthy of critique, in so far as they take from the doctor and give to the organization (e.g., hospitals, private insurers, Medicare), the latter of which then can oversee and direct physician work with greater specificity. They also create fertile conditions for growing the retail philosophy in primary care, a philosophy discussed in Chapter 3. As we will hear, the corporation has a central role in promoting the retail approach due to the latter's need for significant data analytic capabilities, its emphasis on large scale and price competition, and the marketing of variety to customers through "business-to-consumer" offerings that span an array of different service and product areas (Deloitte 2016; Robbins 2016). These forces and their fallout also have consequences for the *relational side* of primary care, as described in Chapter 1, to the extent that they downplay or interfere with doctor-patient interaction; in some cases cheapening complex interpersonal dynamics such as communication, knowledge transfer, listening, trust, empathy, and mutual respect through the misuse of health information technology, emphasis on transactional care efficiency, and overuse of quantification in evaluating appropriate service delivery.

METRIC FEVER IS HERE TO STAY: STANDARDIZING QUALITY AND PAYING FOR VALUE

Metric fever is defined as the intense emphasis within the U.S. health system on measuring, documenting, and reporting a voluminous array of efficiency and quality data that serve as proxies for "good care delivery" and "good health outcomes" and that are increasingly tied to pay-for-performance (P4P) and value-based purchasing (VBP) incentive programs arriving on the scene over the past decade (Centers for Medicare and Medicaid Services 2017; National Committee for Quality Assurance 2016; Rosenthal and Dudley; Wachter 2016). Pay for performance is a payment philosophy that refers generally to different ways that public (e.g., Medicare) and private insurers financially incentivize physicians to meet specific process and outcome metrics addressing care quality, efficiency, and cost. Its widespread use belies its proven lack of efficacy. For example, the use of financial incentives to compensate physicians has received underwhelming support empirically in terms of its effectiveness in improving quality, lowering costs, or inducing long-term behavior change (Eijkenaar et al. 2013; Glickman et al. 2007; Rosenthal and Frank 2006). Many question if it is the best way to motivate professionals like doctors, who in theory are driven in their work more by intrinsic rather than extrinsic rewards (Rosenthal and Frank 2006; Ryan and Deci 2000). Yet, the approach and its underlying Pavlovian philosophy remain appealing to a health policy and management sphere looking for simple answers to complex problems, in this case getting physicians to align their work with the metrics.

Quality improvement is big business in U.S. health care. This movement, led by external accrediting agencies such as the National Committee for Quality Assurance (NCQA); employer-sponsored groups such as the National Quality Forum; and think tanks like the Institute for Healthcare Improvement and Institute of Medicine, has ushered in an age where so-called "experts" from a range of backgrounds dictate the quality rules, through their reputational power (e.g., who would disagree with the Institute of Medicine?) and industry influence. It is a highly institutionalized, ideological environment governed by strict norms regarding how noble goals such as health care quality should be conceptualized, measured, and improved (see Powell and DiMaggio 2012). If quality before was a paternalistic endeavor of "physicians know best," short on precision, transparency, or consistency, it could be said that quality now is an equally paternalistic endeavor of "big employers, insurers, government, and accrediting agencies know best."

"Value-based purchasing" (VBP) is a health care reimbursement approach that uses standardized performance measurement, public reporting of quality data, and new forms of payment such as global budgeting (e.g., a fixed payment for entire groups of patients or services) to improve quality and lower costs (National Business Coalition on Health 2017). Few systematic research findings currently support the approach on a widespread scale, in terms of either significantly lowering care costs or improving quality in transformative ways. Thus, it is a relatively unproven innovation being attempted on a grand scale. Value-based reimbursement implies that physicians and health care organizations like hospitals should have meaningful amounts of their pay tied to demonstrating that they can perform well on a series of standard metrics. These metrics involve numerous quality measures, which may or may not be aggregated into composite "scores," as well as efficiency-related markers that include things like hospital readmission rates, emergency room use, and overuse of expensive imaging tests such as MRIs (magnetic resonance imaging).

A chief goal of value-based purchasing is to limit unpredictability on the payer side associated with a traditional fee-for-service system, which is a "do more get more" system. Value-based purchasing shifts the risk onto those providing care by giving either fixed sums of money, which providers must work efficiently within (or lose money themselves), or incentivized payments that can be obtained by showing that tangible "value-based" outcomes have been met. Medicare is the chief innovator in the VBP movement at the present time, with its goal to soon have over half of all dollars paid out to health care providers tied to showing appropriate performance in several different areas (Centers for Medicare and Medicaid Services 2017).

The Healthcare Effectiveness Data and Information Set (HEDIS) is the poster child for metric fever run wild in health care, forming one of the core foundations for making value-based reimbursement work. Since its advent in the early 1990s, HEDIS has been used to supply performance measures to many pay-for-performance programs, especially those in primary care. HEDIS is a standardized approach to measuring quality. It is so much a part of U.S. health care today even the acronym is copyrighted by the National Committee for Quality Assurance (NCQA), in case there is any question about who owns, administers, and ultimately profits from it. HEDIS looks deceptively simple and benign on the printed page, given that it is a neatly ordered table of measures expressed in short, easy-to-understand statements.

Yet beneath its brevity lay a great deal of administrative and physician work needed to meet its demands (Hoff 2010). It involves almost one hundred separate measures across many areas of primary care delivery, ranging from physician responsibilities to counsel patients in a variety of health care situations (e.g., patients with elevated cholesterol, obesity); to controlling important health markers such as blood pressure and hemoglobin A1C; to conducting medication management for patients; to carefully assessing and monitoring high-risk patients on several indicators (e.g., falls); to providing comprehensive care for patients with chronic diseases such as diabetes. In theory, it sounds good. Who would be against holding physicians accountable for doing more things, rather than less?

But for each primary care physician (PCP), and her or his often understaffed and under-resourced primary care practice, meeting a single HEDIS measure for one's patient population may require a significant amount of time and work; time that the typical PCP may not have in a normal day of 20–30 patient visits, and work which may not value, benefit, or take advantage of the relational aspects of interaction between PCP and patient. Often times, the time and work associated with complying with HEDIS measures involves transactional, process-driven activities that can turn patients into lists of things needing to be done, depending on their symptoms or diagnosis. Most value-based purchasing approaches use HEDIS measures or some variant of them for quality-monitoring in primary care. The typical primary care physician will tell you straight out that just keeping track of all the quality-documentation and reporting demands these insurers make, not even accounting for the clinical care that must be done to fulfill metric requirements, is both frustrating and expensive (Hoff 2010; Hoff, Young, and Collinson 2016).

Increasingly, though, it all must be done to get money back from insurers. For example, in one study done by the author and two colleagues, some Boston-area primary care practices faced unique performance requirements from four or five different major area insurers at once, as well as needing to report additional metrics required by Medicare and Medicaid (Hoff, Young, and Collinson 2016). This same study revealed that many of the physicians in these practices also had meaningful amounts of their annual salaries tied to meeting, documenting, and reporting on different performance measures, sometimes 25 percent or more compensation just from a single insurer. For today's primary care practice, there is no choice in deciding whether or not to meet the expectations of insurers where documenting and reporting quality and efficiency is concerned, and the demands on this front continue to increase (Centers for Medicare and Medicaid Services 2017; Wachter 2016).

The modern-day quality movement in the United States has both benefitted and taken its toll on primary care delivery. Benefitted it in terms of creating more explicit accountability and transparency for physician work, as well as standardizing some needed aspects of care, particularly in areas where diagnosis and treatment is more predictable at times such as in chronic disease care. But one can make a strong case that it has gone too far (Wachter 2016). Before, doctors relied on little but their own word to determine how efficient or high-quality they were in their work. They were the sole determinants of what constituted appropriate diagnostic and treatment pathways (Starr 1982). Too much physician discretion produced unexplained variation, service overuse, and a high-cost system without the commensurate quality outcomes.

In some key ways, things have changed for the better with modern-day quality assessment approaches, especially in basic chronic disease management. For example, there are ways to validate whether a PCP's diabetic patients are receiving necessary tests and having their blood sugar regulated; and it is generally accepted that there exists a single appropriate treatment pathway for diabetics that covers many of their potential health issues. In addition, there are ways of knowing for sure that PCPs are properly screening their patients for debilitating diseases like cancer in timely ways consistent with good, evidence-based prevention. Physicians are held to a standard of care, and must demonstrate they meet that standard.

Generally, there is a proverbial audit trail of work processes and decision points, verified through checklists and reporting systems, to demonstrate which primary care practices and physicians are doing the things needed to achieve select outcomes such as lower hemoglobin A1C's and blood pressure.

Thus, for some patients, metric fever brings with it a level of good, standard care for their particular disease. For insurers and accreditors, the heavy emphasis on documenting and reporting standardized performance across large numbers of physicians makes perfect sense. It allows for relative, useful comparisons of doctors. It simplifies care delivery work in ways that create greater transparency. It provides a more accurate, objective system of verification than simply the physician's own word. It provides a logical use for all the "big data" on patients and their care that is being collected daily now in doctors' offices and hospitals.

Critics disagree. They argue that physician comparisons on standardized performance metrics provide at best a superficial and crude means of determining who provides "good care." They assert that the overuse of metrics encourages gaming and other dysfunctional behavior that undermines doctor-patient trust, as some physicians end up concentrating more on what is being measured, and how to do well on a more narrowly focused band of clinical processes and outcomes (Campbell, McDonald, and Lester 2008; Rosenthal and Frank 2006). In addition, for some standardized measures, such as controlling a diabetic patient's hemoglobin A1C to under 7, or a cholesterol LDL value to under 100, physicians and their staff may feel that they have limited impact on the ultimate outcome. They may believe that patients must shoulder the bulk of the responsibility for improving metrics that are dependent in meaningful part on lifestyle and patient choice. They also may feel that for some patients, the standard benchmarks are not appropriate to aim for or pursue.

The critics fear that metric fever creates adversarial relationships with some patients, and places doctors in a conflict of interest position, namely, needing to show they can get their patients to meet the performance requirements while at the same time respecting their patient's own wishes for self-determination around their health care. Critics also contend that many aspects of good quality care cannot be standardized or fit into a quantifiable metric easily documented and reported, and that these aspects get devalued by physicians over time. Certainly, the more relational, yet proven features of doctor-patient interaction, such as active listening, communication, compassion, asking the right questions, taking a good history and physical, and displaying empathy fit into this category.

All of this, critics conclude, creates a slippery slope into a world where "quality care" is oversimplified for some patients and where good doctoring is reduced to a checklist of "to do's," rather than encompassing a nuanced appreciation for the full range of what a physician does for a given patient at a certain point in time (Wachter 2016). For them, metric fever has taken its toll in subjecting primary care physicians, their staff members, and patients to a complex maze of collecting, documenting, and reporting all sorts of "number-based" medical information; creating a care environment where doing what is needed to "check a box" in the way an insurer or government wants takes precedence over everything else (Hoff, Young, and Collinson 2016).

For example, during the times *live patients* are supposed to be directly interacted with and served, listened to rather than talked at, physicians and their staff members must also concern themselves with acquiring the right kind of quality information from each and every individual; identifying and tracking down noncompliant patients to get the necessary things done for making practice numbers look good; and storing everything in the electronic medical record in predetermined ways preferred by various insurers. Physicians dislike having their work redirected in these ways (Ryan et al. 2015). But they must do it. Besides all the other things a primary care physician's office has to do in a given day, and has had to do for a while, such as get service preauthorizations for patients, coordinate specialist referrals, validate patients' insurance benefits, do prescription refills and ordering, and manage care transitions for patients across hospitals and other doctor offices, all of which consume a fair portion of a PCP's workday (Hoff 2010; The Physicians Foundation 2014), an additional and often unpredictable amount of time and money now is spent on the grunt work of quality metrics.

Another implication of metric fever relates to it supporting new models of payment in primary care such as value-based purchasing. Physicians have to expand their patient panels and have more infrastructure around them to make these reimbursement models work. Their business cannot survive otherwise. For example, the infrastructure needed to document and report on various quality and efficiency measures may involve a highly integrated electronic medical record system in which all staff members must be fluent, costing tens of thousands of dollars and a lot of spare staff time to use as intended. It also includes additional staff time devoted to entering data and tracking down noncompliant patients, as well as obtaining patient information from other providers. Several hours of daily practice capacity are taken up with communications among physicians and staff regarding what tests or exams require doing for which patients, and time for compiling reports and statistics that demonstrate compliance with metric goals. One study supported by the federal government showed that the average annual maintenance cost for data collection and reporting for a single disease, namely, diabetes, was almost $10,000 per practice, after an initial implementation cost of over $15,000 (West et al. 2012). Another survey showed over 60 percent of physicians reporting increased overhead and administrative costs to comply with the Affordable Care Act, the wide-sweeping legislation that has increased the intensity of metric fever in health care (Jackson Healthcare 2015).

A numbers problem also requires attention: To meet the required metrics and show real improvement on a statistically significant or at least population-based scale a physician's office needs larger patient panels, which means a larger number of patients who want to access your office and you as the physician. Patient panels also must grow to maximize the per capita payments associated with bundled or global payment systems that pay prospectively on a per patient basis. Physicians must create appropriate workflows to handle this demand, which forces them into unknown territory (e.g., using teams, electronic medical records, group and virtual visits with patients) and things they generally are not good at (e.g., being managers, involving themselves in business decisions). Having to expand the number of patients in a practice makes everyday work life much more complex for the doctor, reduces relational care provision to a luxury, and can create a general form of angst toward patients who become less differentiated, given that many are known less well and seen less often. The levels of time and energy, and likely sacrifice of pay, to develop deeper, extended relationships with even a subset of individual patients can loom as a chore rather than an opportunity. It also may not be something for which the physician gets financially rewarded, as patient quantity begins to count more than quality.

THE HEAVY BURDEN OF THE
PATIENT-CENTERED MEDICAL HOME

As discussed earlier, the quality expectations embedded in value-based purchasing approaches create massive administrative expectations for primary care physicians, taking already squeezed workdays and threatening to turn physician attention away from individual patient relationships toward those with insurers and *patient populations* with similar diseases. The largest initiative in primary care of the past decade is reflective of many of these dynamics, as well as the perils of metric fever gone wild. It is called the *patient-centered medical home* (PCMH). At a general level, the PCMH is a philosophy of how primary care practices should think of themselves—that is, as a sort of "one-stop shop" for any and all primary care services, with the PCP the grand coordinator of care. In reality, however, the PCMH has remained a vague, quixotic concept implemented through a long checklist of metrics across various areas of office and clinical work. No primary care practice in the United States can call itself a "medical home" without gaining the official seal of approval from the National Committee for Quality Assurance (NCQA), the most important quality accreditation organization for ambulatory care in the country (NCQA 2015).

Practices seeking to acquire and keep medical home accreditation must agree to pay attention to, document, and track and report regularly on dozens of metrics that speak to whether they have in place the workflows, office policies, and care protocols that the NCQA deems appropriate. Most quality measurement for the medical home originates with the question, "Can a primary care practice show it has certain things in place?" This approach emphasizes what the "home" looks like structurally inside and out, that is, the look of its siding, paint job, and furniture—rather than the experience of how people actually live in it on a daily basis. Its appealing name initially sucked in primary care physicians desperate for greater attention paid to their craft. Many of those physicians now see it as both a burden and a bait and switch perpetrated on their practices (The Physicians Foundation 2014).

In return for this PCMH "Good Housekeeping seal of approval" from NCQA, some primary care practices receive additional reimbursement from insurers and government in the form of "care management" fees paid on the basis of the total number of patients in the practice; enhanced payments for doing certain types of service delivery in a consistent fashion; or extra dollars for things like maintaining particular types of functionality with the use of the electronic health record. Many primary care practices, however, do not see any new financial gain by meeting the requirements for medical home accreditation. Rather, they are expected to meet the standards and maintain all the proof of doing so as an addition to their everyday patient care activities. Or, if an insurer or government does throw them a few extra dollars, they will tell you those dollars are eaten up quickly with the added costs of trying to put everything in place to meet the performance standard.

This is the sneaky aspect of the model. It has forced primary care physicians to bend more to the will of insurers or risk being branded as outliers among their peers, and suffer reimbursement problems in the process. In short, they have little choice but to go along. Through this checklist-based verification process, done through a combination of self-reporting and periodic audits, primary care practices demonstrate to the outside world that they have "met the PCMH standard," which then gets them into the club, although as a lot of prior research shows, getting into the club does not always guarantee significantly better patient care, patient experiences, or doctor-patient relationships (Hoff 2013; Hoff, Weller, and DePuccio 2012; Jackson et al. 2013; Werner et al. 2013). The medical home model has required a tremendous amount of financial investment, time, and physician energy. Yet the overall results are modest at best. Just look at a recent report from a reputable health care foundation to understand how convoluted and sketchy the medical home evaluation results being reported out are—this report spends more time trying to justify the design flaws in current medical home demonstration projects and in the end simply states that the PCMH evaluations they looked at are likely overstating results or cannot report out results with any confidence (Nielsen et al. 2016). Caveat emptor.

The PCMH model feeds into the corporate umbrella overseeing primary care, so there is a motive on the part of large health care delivery organizations to support and control the medical home effort. For example, new, highly paid staff, such as quality improvement directors and "big data" analysts; entire departments resourced to do quality and performance management; large investments in health information technology and patient data registries—an entire hidden industry within primary care is devoted solely to making primary care physicians and their practices look good to insurers and government agencies on aspects of medical home care. This allows health care organizations to grow ever larger, particularly on the administrative side, and takes sparse dollars out of the doctor's hands that could be used to subsidize longer office visits, or more time spent in direct interaction with patients building relational features. It also justifies large investments in electronic medical records, which are positioned as the tools that can make a model like the PCMH work. This hidden industry affects doctors and their work in potentially negative ways for relational care.

The PCMH model in primary care has not proven to be the panacea to U.S. primary care ills, or the reinvention of a physician-centric model of care. Although one of its principles is a "personal physician" for every patient, there is, in fact, little evidence showing that the PCMH has produced better doctor-patient relationships, or improved the relational aspects of care (e.g., trust) very much. That said, the medical home designation does confer a form of external legitimacy on primary care physicians; legitimacy that remains perhaps their last best claim to being afforded special dispensation as the central figures in U.S. primary care medicine. But the underperformance of this model, and its preoccupation with guideline-driven care, raise the question of why we continue to invest so much time, money, and energy in it.

Still, to some the medical home initiative remains appealing in the abstract, that is, a set of metrics and standards focused on trying to make primary care more orderly, systematic, and perhaps even "patient-centered" from the perspective of: (a) making sure certain appropriate things get done; (b) practices move into the 21st century in their use of information technology; and (c) various forms of basic communication (e.g., clinical visit summaries for patients) are embedded into everyday practice in a consistent way. Yet, actually fulfilling the spirit and not simply the letter of medical home requirements, which means becoming a place where patients get the full attention of their personal physician and are treated with a healthy respect for all their unique needs, is more elusive. Another danger with the medical home innovation is that the focus on "checking the medical home boxes" forces doctors and their staff members into a world where patients become standardized widgets, who are thought about similarly, and from whom the same metric-related information must be extracted at every possible turn. I have seen this in my own research on medical home implementation (Hoff 2013; Hoff and DePuccio 2016; Hoff and Scott 2016).

Physicians remain skeptical. Only one-third of primary care physicians recently surveyed nationally felt that the medical home model of care had a positive impact on the quality of care for patients. The remaining two-thirds felt it had either no impact, a negative impact, or were not sure whether it had any impact at all (Ryan et al. 2015). Primary care physicians in another large national survey were underwhelmed by the medical home model of care; 38 percent felt that the model was unlikely to either improve quality or reduce costs, and another 20 percent were unsure about the structure and purpose of the model (The Physicians Foundation 2014). That's a lot of ambivalence for such an appealing innovation on paper, particularly from those individuals (aside from patients) who should be jumping up and down the most for it, given its marketing pitch as a doctor-patient relationship enhancement tool. Coupled with its less than stellar results, one wonders if the medical home model is another in a long line of policy interventions (e.g., capitation, managed care, safety reporting systems) that people cling to because they sweep complex problems under the rug, and lay a soft, warm blanket of simplicity over the hard realities of what it will take to fix U.S. primary care—allowing policy makers, consultants, software vendors, and accrediting agencies to sleep better at night, but not the two parties (doctors and patients) who really count.

THE CORPORATE, TIGHTLY MANAGED UMBRELLA OVERSEEING TODAY'S PRIMARY CARE

The quality and value-based purchasing movements also have been accompanied in primary care by the increasing shift of primary care physicians into salaried employment, often in larger organizations with the resources and administrative expertise to manage financial risk, monitor quality, and invest in needed infrastructure (Rosenthal 2014). Over half of primary care physicians now work as salaried employees, and the vast majority of those newly hired are employees (Singleton and Miller 2015). In fact, finding many young PCPs who want to buy into a practice early in their career might prove to be quite an Easter egg hunt. Young physicians especially eschew taking on the business pressures and administrative responsibilities that come with a self-employed career, preferring work schedules and career burdens that allow them to maintain a sizeable commitment to nonwork activities (Hoff and Pohl 2017). Thus, most of them choose salaried employment (Hoff 2010; The Physicians Foundation 2014).

Prior to the advent of health care reform in the United States, most physicians already stated that their practices were overextended with too many patients and not enough administrative support or resources for handling the voluminous requirements of quality improvement activities (The Physicians Foundation 2008). The Affordable Care Act (ACA) and more recently Medicare's VPB program called the Medicare Access and CHIP Reauthorization Act (MACRA) only add to that feeling (Jackson Healthcare 2015; The Physicians Foundation 2014). The ACA, through its focus on the creation of big structures such as Accountable Care Organizations, combined with the desire to move reimbursement more into fixed amounts or bundles, force the industry to take a "bigger is better" mentality in making value-based payment pay.

For instance, with payment that involves a fixed amount per a given patient population, enough dollars need to be captured per patient in that particular population to justify the significant financial investments in information technology, staffing, and business expertise physician offices must make for being good at the quality game, which is necessary for getting these dollars in the first place, and then for getting even more payment down the road. As noted earlier, a certain level of scale is necessary to do things such as manage risk in specific patient populations (e.g., diabetics, hypertensives); ensure all needed tests and screens are being done on certain patients in a timely manner; and identifying, through the use of data analytics, which patients are noncompliant and thus likely to skew various quality metrics for the office in ways that could jeopardize payment.

Physicians who become employees understand this reality. It leaves many of the older ones, who are accustomed to a smaller, more independent world of private practice, increasingly miserable (The Physicians Foundation 2014). But they also realize there is little choice. Primary care physicians especially have to align themselves with bigger administrative structures to gain negotiating leverage and access to resources that help them manage their practices. As a result, primary care practices have recently made up the largest portion of acquisitions by hospitals (Jackson Healthcare 2015). Some of these structures are supported by private capital that seeks its own return on investment through the creation of efficient, metric-skilled primary care practice organizations that can then be sold to larger care systems and insurers (Kutscher 2015).

The larger administrative organizations that many physicians have signed onto in seeking cover from the tsunami of metrics, documentation, and reporting described above gain control over doctor-patient relationships as they become direct physician employers or de facto employers by virtue of how the individual physician must rely upon them. Physicians give up a tremendous degree of control to these structures, even if they technically "own them" in some instances, and they acquiesce to abide by the larger organizational policies and work requirements the organizations mandate. In two of my research projects, a number of the primary care practices participating in each project voluntarily joined a "physician-driven" administrative organization that was funded by investments each of the practices made. Physicians in these structures handed over substantial power to the organization; for example, in areas such as negotiating reimbursement contracts with insurers; defining the types of performance metrics and financial incentives for physicians to work under; and workload targets. They allowed these larger organizations to make important decisions related to patient care; decisions that in some cases overrode individual physician preferences.

Of course, this trend is less of a problem for some and instead presents an opportunity for enhancing the relationships patients have with *the health system* as an entity. It provides fertile ground for retail strategies and tactics that rely less on physician brand and more on organizational brand to enter the health care marketplace. For example, having larger organizations assume control over patient care workflows, quality improvement

policies, and personnel management gives them an opportunity to connect directly with the individual patient. It allows these organizations to
cultivate their own image as patient advocates. It lets them broaden their
perceived usefulness for patients beyond direct care delivery and into
other walks of life that might include non-health care related services. As a
result, it also offers the potential for other buying and engagement opportunities with patients. For these reasons, hospitals and larger care delivery systems, especially those with locally and nationally reputable names,
such as Cleveland Clinic or Mayo, desire to make a direct investment in
primary care physicians and their office practices.

Still, the implications of this transfer of roles from individual physician
to the corporate organization is profound. It allows the latter to mediate
between doctor and patient in ways that arguably weaken the physician's
legitimacy over patient care. For example, as the organization enforces
clinical policies that require all patients with certain characteristics or
disease states to receive specific tests or care, regardless of whether the
physician or patient (or both) feel such tests or care are appropriate in a
given case, physician-patient relationships may become strained. A colonoscopy for a patient over age 50 is mandated as "good care" by insurers
but some over-50 patients may not want to have a colonoscopy. For some
patients with low-risk profiles, it may not be truly necessary to have one
done immediately at age 50. Yet, under modern reimbursement systems
and insurer quality guidelines, physicians could be penalized for patients
who exhibit personal preferences other than what a clinical guideline
states. Consequently, physicians may come to view certain patients in
negative ways that undermine their ability to be their patient's advocate.
At the same time, patients may misconstrue physician behavior and feel
pressured to get a certain test or screening performed, even if they (the
patients) do not want it done. Doctors may get angry at some of their
patients for being recalcitrant in getting care, particularly those who, for
whatever reason, do not or cannot fall in line with what the quality metrics
require. Doctor-patient relationships suffer.

In addition, this transfer of roles from doctor to organization shapes
how work is organized in primary care. For instance, if corporate directives stemming from how to best manage fixed pots of reimbursement
include specifying how many patients physicians must see in a day, or

which particular quality metrics must be met to the letter and by when, and individual compensation is tied to these things, physician practices are forced to structure workflow in ways that pay close attention to maximizing what it is the organization wants, and not necessarily to meet the relational care goals between doctors and their patients. Thus, office visits may be shorter; the electronic medical record grows more intrusive; non-physician staff may more frequently substitute in certain activities with patients that used to involve physicians; patients will get to see their regular physician less; and physicians may spend more exam room time interacting strategically with patients around particular aspects of their care rather than engaging in proactive listening, letting patients tell their stories, and investigating the unknown (Hoff 2010).

Perhaps the organizational structure gaining the most attention these days is the Accountable Care Organization (ACO); a structure that comes directly from the Affordable Care Act. According to some, ACOs are the next best thing in health care organizational innovation, and they have implications for primary care. On paper, ACOs are designed as integrated care delivery systems, involving both primary and specialty care, and sometimes other care such as home health. The players within an ACO share the financial risk for care delivered within that system. They earn profit in different but related ways: by not spending all the dollars they are given, by meeting specific quality improvement and cost reduction targets and earning incentives, and by receiving additional funds each budget year to the extent they have demonstrated the kinds of care delivery insurers want (Gold 2011).

Approximately 24 million covered lives are now in ACOs nationally, and estimates for the near future triple that number (Muhlestein 2015). The number of commercial insurers involved in ACO contracting is increasing steadily over time. Medicare and Medicaid are enthusiastically embracing the model in their quest to move toward global payment that shifts greater risk onto physicians and hospitals (Muhlestein 2015). Medicare has committed to providing 50 percent or more of its payouts through value-based mechanisms, and ACOs are thought to be a big part of making that approach successful.

What being in an ACO means for the doctor-patient relationship in primary care is not thought about much by policy makers or managers now pushing this structure, but its impact is both subtle and profound. Consider the underlying logic of the ACO structure itself. First, an ACO consists of organizations and professionals that *provide the care to patients.* At the same time, however, by taking on more of the financial risk in caring for a patient population, an ACO also has to think *like an insurance company.* In this dual role, where potential conflicts of interest abound, the ACO has to accomplish certain goals. First, it must create certain everyday efficiencies in how care is delivered. These efficiencies, some of which have been mentioned above, have at their center the removal of the physician from aspects of care delivery that do not provide enough revenue or value to cover the physician's cost. Where technology and lower-cost staff can be substituted into workflows, they are in ways that further remove patients from contact with their doctor.

The ACO also needs its primary care physicians to aggressively manage certain types of patients of higher cost to the system of care within the ACO, that is, patients who inevitably burn dollars through overuse or not engaging enough in prevention. Otherwise, the ACO may lose financial incentives that are linked to specific population health outcomes, or simply have its profit margin squeezed for the pot of dollars it already has been given, by disproportionately providing too many services to particular patients on the back end. In an ACO environment, too many unmanageable chronic disease patients become money losers for the organization within a global payment sphere. The business model of an ACO, coupled with a value-based reimbursement formula, places the primary care physician at the center of controlling preventable costs and making sure that existing quality, particularly with respect to chronic disease patients, meets the preferred targets set by the entities funding the ACO.

ACOs generally do not offer a financial windfall for primary care physicians. Instead, it may resemble a shell game, moving dollars that were provided to PCPs through a fee-for-service system into a riskier (for PCPs) arrangement wherein doctors must demonstrate they are hitting the quality and efficiency targets set for them. Given both limited resources and capacity issues within all primary care settings that continue unabated (Jackson Healthcare 2015), this forces PCPs to make choices around how to use their limited time (Hoff 2010). Thinking like a PCP offers insights in this regard: Do I spend my workday seeing relatively healthy patients for whom I receive few extra dollars? Or do I spend valuable time getting the sicker or noncompliant patients in front of me, because it is those patients who directly affect my quality scores, cost efficiency (e.g., visits to emergency rooms and hospitals) and, as a result, increasingly bigger chunks of my salary?

Do I focus on low-margin, fee-for-service medicine, taking care of coughs and sniffles, or do I let someone else take over that work, instead trying to fill my visit slots with annual physicals, Medicare follow-ups, and *complex* chronic disease management, all of which bring me either fee-for-service revenue or good incentive dollars? Do I even deal with things like mental health, for which I do not get paid formally and which also open up Pandora's boxes full of additional uncompensated care coordination on my part for some of my patients? Do I need to limit my time interacting with any given patient, because it is not the length of my interaction with patients that is financially rewarded? Questions like this are problematic for primary care physicians to have to ask themselves, in large part because they create an air of ambiguity in their work with patients. Their answers also decide choices for physicians around which types of patients get ongoing relationships with them, which do not, and how those relationships will look in terms of time and attention.

THE NEED FOR ACCESS AND CORPORATE AMBIVALENCE TO RELATIONAL CARE

The Affordable Care Act's expansion of health insurance, the aging of the U.S. population, and the continued shortage of PCPs nationally have combined to make access to primary care the key issue now across the United States. Many parts of the country suffer from shortages in physicians, particularly in primary care (Health Resources and Services Administration 2017). There are over 6,000 primary care shortage areas in the United States (Health Resources and Services Administration 2016). This staggering figure runs up against the upwards of 20 million people who have become newly insured in the United States since 2008 (Department of Health and Human Services 2016). Without a doubt, such insurance expansion has placed enormous strains on an already inadequate primary care system in the United States. These strains involve longer wait times to see primary care doctors; longer distances that must be travelled to get primary care in some parts of the country; and an increased disease burden going into doctors' offices, making it difficult for primary care physicians to slow down their daily work treadmills and spend more time getting to know their newer patients.

For example, in Massachusetts, where I live, approximately 96 percent of citizens are insured. That said, upon first moving to the Boston area several years ago my family members and I had to wait five months to get new patient appointments with primary care physicians from the largest, most renowned health care system in Boston. Generally, wait times in Boston to see a family physician are on average 66 days, and they range from a low of 12 days to a high of 152 days (Merritt Hawkins 2014). In 10 of the 15 largest U.S. cities, new patient wait times in family practice increased between 2009 and 2013, with some average wait times going up significantly in large urban markets such as Philadelphia, Atlanta, Portland, and Seattle (Merritt Hawkins 2014). Now these statistics are only for a new patient appointment and physical. They do not speak to the reality of how difficult it has become to see your assigned primary care physician on a regular basis, that is, outside of the once a year checkups allowed through Obamacare and your insurance plan. Over 40 percent of respondents in a recent national patient survey stated that they do not always get timely appointments, care, and information from their primary care physicians (Agency for Healthcare Research and Quality 2015).

The provision of insurance to millions of additional citizens in the United States means that the demands on primary care grow. Already, half a billion ambulatory care visits per year are conducted in the United States (Centers for Disease Control and Prevention 2014). The provisions in the Affordable Care Act that allow individuals to obtain free preventive screenings and checkups add to the primary care physician visit burden. The increasing morbidity of the population, particularly seniors who have multiple chronic diseases, also makes primary care work for some individuals difficult and time consuming to do. The over-65 population is increasing dramatically in the United States, and this population suffers from higher rates of chronic disease and co-occurring chronic diseases than any other cohort (Centers for Disease Control and Prevention 2017). Add to that the unpredictable nature of primary care medicine, in which patients often present with hidden, time-intensive issues such as depression, and where there is much less routine in how primary care physicians do their work than we might imagine (Hoff 2010).

While demand grows, primary care physician supply does not. There is consensus that a primary care physician shortage will exist in the near future, and shortfalls are predicted to upwards of 30,000 PCPs nationally by 2025 (Association of American Medical Colleges [AAMC] 2015). Despite the rhetoric about how to get more medical students to choose a primary care field, the reality is that there will be far too few of them to handle the patient care requirements of a larger, aging, and more insured population. Physician supply generally will not be able to meet the expected patient demand, with upwards of 90,000 additional physicians, primary care and specialists, required by 2025 (AAMC 2015).

Into this access void steps the growth of disruptive innovations, particularly in primary care, designed to get patients into cheaper, less relational forms of care delivery. One of these innovations is retail clinics—a fast food version of primary care in which patients are offered a limited buffet of services, mostly addressing low-level acute care issues, and which use non-physician providers such as nurse practitioners to interact with patients (Hwang and Mehrotra 2013). Retail clinics undermine the doctor-patient relationship in primary care because they do not employ physicians or emphasize care continuity with the same provider over time. The number of retail clinics remains small nationally, increasing from 200 to over 1,800 between 2006 and 2014, accounting for over 10 million primary care visits in the United States (Jaspen 2016). Owned and operated chiefly by corporations such as CVSHealth and Walgreens, as well as by hospital systems, retail clinics offer no repeat care (you normally cannot return for the same issue twice), no complex care, and no ability to treat the entire patient in a holistic manner.

However, these outlets fill a niche because they allow greater convenience for individuals who value it, and the small body of research that exists shows they can do basic clinical jobs fairly well, despite not necessarily saving the system any real dollars (Ashwood et al. 2016). For all their hype, retail clinics remain a work in progress, and an unproven transformative disruption for the U.S. health care industry. What they do signal, though, is a strong desire on the part of industry stakeholders and venture capitalists to bring retail thinking into health care, driving a further wedge between doctor and patient through strategic actions designed to have the larger organization gain the patient's loyalty and trust, largely at the expense of individual physicians. If you go to a Minute Clinic, you are a CVSHealth patient, not a particular doctor's patient.

In a similar vein, urgent care centers (Creswell 2014) are popping up across the country, supported in no small part by private equity interests looking to make a profit. Unlike retail clinics, this delivery innovation often employs physicians, and may, in fact, be owned and operated by a physician group (Urgent Care Association of America 2017). There are 7,100 urgent care centers nationally, providing a range of services (Urgent Care Association of America [UCAoA] 2017). Approximately 20 percent of these centers belong to larger systems, putting a lot of urgent care in the hands of very large corporations. Urgent care centers often are highlighted as promising areas for venture capital investment, with one media outlet reporting that "despite a decrease in the number of urgent care clinics as of late, investors have pumped roughly $3 billion into the burgeoning urgent care industry since 2008" (Becker et al. 2016). Larger hospital systems also are expanding into the urgent care center business, as are specialty areas such as orthopedics (Becker et al. 2016).

Urgent care centers fill an important access gap by providing after-hours, acute care access for patients. Weekend hours, nightly hours, no appointment needed, the ability to diagnosis and treat more complex acute conditions—this is what makes them an appealing option for the general public. I have been to plenty of urgent care centers, and they have provided value to me with respect to convenience and timely access. That said, by virtue of how they are staffed and run, urgent care centers are not interested in creating strong doctor-patient relationships, or engaging in time-consuming, more relational service delivery involving chronic disease management, prevention, and behavioral health. Urgent care centers are meant to generate a high volume of low-margin yet simple patient care transactions that yield profit for investors and serve as "loss leaders" for retail outlets, hospitals, and pharmacy chains—giving patients a convenient way to bring their health and non-health care business to them rather than to a competitor.

Staffing at urgent care centers is an example of an operational decision done more in the name of transactional care than strong doctor-patient relationships. According to the UCAoA:

> The majority of urgent care centers use a 'physician-based' model, typically using family practice physicians and emergency physicians. . . . More and more, urgent care centers also staff with physician assistants and sometimes nurse practitioners. There is no 'recommended' or 'standard' or 'perfect' staffing model. This is determined individually by each center and varies depending on the philosophy of the center, the local labor market, scope of practice, state practice laws, and the like. (UCAoA 2016)

This general statement implies lots of variation across the country relative to the types of professional-patient interactions one will find. What it does make clear is that the potential for a patient to move through urgent care centers and develop an ongoing relationship with the same physician that is consistent and lasts over time are slim. Urgent care centers tend to use lots of "moonlighting" doctors who work on a contractual basis staffing a center one or two days a week for extra compensation (as they normally have one or more clinical jobs elsewhere), and increasingly use non-physician providers because they cost less and improve margins. Referred to in the 1980s as a "doc in a box," urgent care centers remain best defined as episodic sources of quick and lower-cost emergency care, done at one's leisure. They relieve the strain on emergency rooms, while also allowing today's PCPs to work a nine-to-five schedule free of guilt and obligation. But they represent a further development on the road to weakened doctor-patient relationships in U.S. health care. They teach patients a very different lesson about what should be valued in their care delivery, namely convenience and quick service over strong interpersonal connections and the features associated with it (e.g., trust, communication, listening).

Finally, there is the disruptive potential of technology to help alleviate the access problems now encountered in the U.S. health system. I say potential because there is still much to question about the future of technology in care delivery. Certainly, web- and app-based services such as

ZocDoc and Doctor on Demand, among others, address the primary care access issue by offering "real-time" opportunities for patients to get expert clinical advice on problems and symptoms. ZocDoc, a hybrid of "Yelp!" and "Open Table" approaches to scheduling physician visits and seeing patient ratings of doctors, has been a fast-growing service catering to those living in areas with a requisite supply of physicians and patients interested in convenience above all else. With ZocDoc, one may get plugged into a very good physician, only that physician performs in the same capacity as the urgent care center—providing episodic interactions that focus on the immediate symptoms or complaint, and which do not produce continuous care over time (unless the physician is taking new patients and the initial visit leads to the physician willing to take the patient on their existing panel of patients). ITriage is a mobile app meant to connect individuals more closely to their health care, seek out advice on their symptoms, and help them to locate physicians in their area. Some apps like Doctor on Demand also will, for a fee, allow patients to connect with physicians through the app, get advice on their condition, and receive initial treatment options.

All of this technology has had slower uptake among patients than technology pundits or the entrepreneurs driving these innovations would like, although it is fair to take a longer-term perspective here and note that most patients have had little ability to drive their own health care in the past, so it is not surprising that tools that increase patient ability to do so may take a while to be adopted. That said, technologies such as wearables, mobile health apps, and even electronic health records have underwhelmed in their ability to enhance the patient experience or improve key aspects of health care, such as quality or efficiency (Chaudhry et al. 2006; Free et al. 2013; Endeavour Partners 2014; Lehman 2015). Again, though, it is not the short-term success of a given health care technology that is the important focus here. Rather, it is the reality that much of this technology serves as a profit, brand, or market-share enhancing vehicle for investors or companies. For example, ITriage is owned by an insurance company, Aetna, which wants to use ITriage to enhance its reputational value among patients; push models such as patient self-management, which are good for its own core insurance business; broaden product lines to gain additional profit and shareholder value as a corporation; and perhaps potentially gain greater control in a marketplace that is integrating the insurance and care delivery sides of the business.

If anything, the need for better access to care in the United States, combined with physician shortfalls, upends existing logics within the system that have guided its evolution over the past 50 years, with much of those logics orbiting around the central idea that the doctor-patient relationship matters greatly, face-to-face care matters, and that patients must see their personal physicians over time to get good health care. In many ways, the access problem now trumps the quality problem in the United States, at least in the short term. Solving this problem produces a sustained *transactional* innovation focus in the industry. Combine this reality with years of an increasingly dumbed-down, overly standardized, and distinctly non-interpersonal approach to improving care quality, and it becomes clear that an intellectual void exists within the system for how to frame what patients need and want; a void that creates opportunity for alternative logics to gain traction. Among those logics are consumerism and retail thinking—influential ideas that have transformed the American way of life across other industries and which now view health care delivery as the next bastion with which to reshape how people think and behave.

Chapter 3

Retail Thinking Comes to Health Care

The Patient as Consumer

U.S. health care is in a state of flux regarding how to think about patients, and how best to connect with them in the system. A single dominant ideology for how to deliver care or create value for patients does not exist at present. But the on-the-ground conditions described favor the entrance of retail thinking into health care. Much of the venture capital moving into health care from outside the industry is betting on a transformational shift in the way this sector functions, toward business models that involve patients as proactive shoppers interested in innovations that make their health care experience more affordable, accessible, and convenient (Booz and Co. 2008). The external forces described in the prior chapter create a perfect storm, in which a next logical chain of developments involve the health care marketplace seeking to turn patients into "consumers." Here is a concise definition of the retail philosophy:

> Retail is the process of selling consumer goods and/or services to customers through multiple channels of distribution to earn a profit. Demand is created through diverse target markets and promotional tactics, satisfying consumers' wants and needs through a lean supply chain. (Wikipedia, 2017, https://en.wikipedia.org/wiki/Retail)

This definition summarizes the retail philosophy. More than anything else, retail is about *selling* things, whether tangible (e.g., a toaster) or intangible (e.g., good service; a relaxing vacation experience). It is also about purchasers *consuming* those things they do buy, with the idea that if the consumption experience is a satisfying one, they will want or require more of those things in the future. Through the consumer lens, all relational roads between buyer and seller must lead to the purchasing goal to justify the retail approach in all its strategic and tactical forms. The top retailers nationally include Walmart, Target, Home Depot, and Amazon—companies whose very existence centers on selling products to individuals and developing *purchasing relationships* with buyers that lead to repeat business (National Retail Federation 2015). Also on the top ten list of retail companies are the two major pharmacy chains, CVS Caremark and Walgreens, both in the business of health care (traditionally pharmaceuticals) but who first and foremost have a mission to create strong buyer-seller relationships with consumers around a wide range of health and beauty products.

These buyer-seller relationships do not manifest as interpersonal (between people) but rather between company and consumer. This makes them different and more artificial in nature. The currency that builds and sustains such relationships does not consist of social exchange or emotional connections between individuals. Instead, it involves the stability and reliability of purchase transactions accumulated over time. The mutual interdependency presumed to exist in a strong doctor-patient relationship, where each party provides the other with intangible rewards, for example, in the doctor's case, professional satisfaction and fulfillment and, in the patient's case, healing and emotional bonding, is absent in retail relationships. It is absent because the organization itself is not human, that is, it has no personality, no ability to feel or express emotion, and no ability to relate on an interpersonal level with the individual.

Although patients do purchase services from their physicians and thus perform within the context of a type of buyer-seller relationship, through the act of seeking them out for help, the acts of selling or purchasing the service are not intended as the sine qua non of the dyadic interaction, and they are not the chief outcomes of interest for either party. Rather, it is in maximizing the relational features of social exchange where the most value is ultimately created for both doctor and patient. Getting helped; being trusted and feeling trust; feeling comforted; having someone listen and express empathy; gaining emotional support; being able to provide help, comfort, and compassion to another human being seeking your guidance—these features are the ultimate things of value sought by each party to the relationship. The retail philosophy may seek in its own way to recreate some of this more *organic* interpersonal currency, but its treatment of health care as a commodity must pursue impersonal, mechanical actions that involve getting to know patients distally through big data; aggregating individuals into homogenous subgroups of similar wants and needs; and then attempting, through marketing messages and efficient distribution efforts to get those subgroups acting in ways that produce a profit-oriented benefit for the organization. These actions, if done right, enhance the future prospects of even more transactions between the two entities.

Retail approaches rely more upon transactional rather than relational exchanges between buyer and seller (see Table 3.1). The differences between the two forms of exchange are profound. Essentially, transactional exchanges are ritualized and highly discrete; focused on meeting prespecified, explicit obligations of an economic nature between buyer and seller. Relational exchanges may involve varied and customized obligations; are ongoing and interpersonal; involve shared benefits between buyer and seller; and aim for noneconomic forms of reward. Their interpersonal and socially constructed nature also makes relational exchanges more likely to produce the type of trust between entities, as described in Chapter 1, that is seen as integral to an effective doctor-patient relationship, and which is furthered through important dynamics such as communication, compassion, listening, and empathy.

Sectors that use the retail approach with success include automobiles, food and beverage, fashion, banking, hospitality, travel, and media and broadcasting. As the definition above also states, another reason why companies use a retail approach is to *earn a profit*. This is the primary reason companies such as Amazon, Walmart, Google, and a variety of start-ups funded with private investor money will enter the health care space. The retail approach is not a philosophy or set of tools whose implicit nature is benevolence relative to the individuals targeted for selling purposes. Its inherent nature is not to achieve equity, fairness, or social justice in its drive to sell things to people. It is a way of thinking aligned with the idea of a *marketplace*. As such, it consists of a philosophy and set of tools intended to "create demand" within a group of like-minded individuals with the

Table 3.1 COMPARISON OF TRANSACTIONAL VERSUS
RELATIONAL EXCHANGES

Transactional Exchange	Relational Exchange
Short-duration exchanges, distinct beginning and end points	Longer duration exchanges, reflects ongoing process of an interpersonal nature
Standardized, explicit obligations	Customized obligations arising from prior interactions between relationship parties
Lower uncertainty leading to exchange stability; more predictable	Higher uncertainty leading to some exchange instability; less predictable
Minimal personal relationships involved	Personal relationships involved
No expectation of future exchange per se	Expectation of ongoing future interactions
Economic satisfaction dominant, explicit rewards and focus on standardizing "value transmission" to groups of purchasers	Noneconomic satisfaction important, intangible as well as explicit rewards; "value" more tailored to individual and less clear at times during single exchanges
Ritualistic, prespecified communications between buyer and seller; heavy emphasis on marketing and "brand selling"	Little emphasis on marketing or preplanned communications; more informal and emergent value creation that becomes "self-evident" to relationship parties

goal of having those individuals see value in some service or product an organization offers, and then obtain that service or product, as well as others, through transactional exchanges. In short, retail is focused on *monetizing* buyer-seller relationships (Booz and Co. 2008).

This is a critical set of points to appreciate when we discuss the role of retail in our health care system. On paper there are tangible reasons why the U.S. health care system would consider adopting the retail approach more heavily in its business models. But there is no ambiguity in the ultimate goals of employing such an approach. *Selling things* (e.g., products, services, ways of thinking) and *earning a profit* occupy the interests of those who employ retail methods, regardless of whether they are a "big-box" store, technology company, hospital, physician office, insurer, airline, or car dealership. Thus, "wellness" innovations such as fitness watches and calorie tracking apps that are marketed and sold using a retail philosophy do not have as their first motivation decreasing the level of obesity in American society, or making individuals healthier as an end unto itself.

Such innovations are meant primarily to make (or save) money for some organization, enhance an organization's brand, or grow loyal customers for the companies pushing them. This corporate self-interest comes first, and any positive health-related benefit for individuals or society second. If the two separate goals converge, all the better for both parties to the transactions, but it is organizational self-interest that seeks to win the day in an either-or situation. A subtle point perhaps, but one important to keep in mind because it raises ethical questions related to what we want a health care system to do for us and who we want doing it. It also calls out retail-oriented organizations in terms of how beholden they would be to money-losing or profit-neutral health care innovations that also improve care in tangible ways for the patient.

For the U.S. health care industry, the retail philosophy and its tools have an appealing face validity for offering potential improvements across the board for patients. For example, the joke I often use with my health care students is that the way U.S. health care organizations have traditionally defined the "4 P's," a key focus of retail thinking, has been: Product: whatever it is we want to sell to you; Price: whatever we can charge; Promotion: what promotion, just take what we give you, and you'll like it; and Place: you come to us, we don't come to you. Of course, this joke has often times been all too real for us as patients when it comes to how we use and experience the system. Retail thinking might change some of this negative reality for the better.

For example, by focusing more sharply on a variety of patien
wants, and expectations, even if for the main goal of selling them things—
the system would have to change the ways it conducts business in fundamental ways. Some of these changes would produce enormous benefits
and greater leverage for patients, particularly in a world of high-deductible
health plans and greater out-of-pocket expenses. In an increasing number and variety of situations, organizations would *listen* to patients, then
take that information and craft services and products in ways that patients
would find do, indeed, match some of what they need, want, or prefer.
Thus, for example, if patients are sick and tired of not gaining timely access
to their primary care doctor, retail thinking may hear that frustration and
push innovation that gives those patients new access points for primary
care built first and foremost around the goal of timely access and convenience. In fact, that is now happening.

In addition, the general idea of "consumer activation" would be appro-
priated by some health care organizations to mean "patient activation" in
the clinical sense, and this could spur innovation in important areas ripe
for continued service enhancements, such as patient self-management,
chronic disease management, insurance purchasing, and preventive medicine. A retail-thinking sector competing more on the basis of price and
efficiency could produce lower prices for some things, create a range of different services and products for patients based on varying levels of afford-
ability, and improve people's access to needed services such as primary
care. The emphasis on simplicity in all its forms, theoretically part of the
consumer-focused mantra, could translate for patients into a health care
marketplace that provides them greater transparency with respect to how
much things cost and from which organizations to purchase them. Finally,
having health care companies take an interest in controlling as much of
the upstream and downstream value chain around their products as possible might reduce service fragmentation and create greater accountability;
for instance, an insurance plan might work alongside a hospital system to
identify and solve issues for their customers not just around insurance but
also around other parts of the care delivery continuum.

On the down side, pursuing a retail philosophy within the industry brings with it a host of meaningful risks for patients and their care.
These include the loss of privacy and personal control related to sensitive

health information that organizations need to segment populations and create selling opportunities; decreased focus on individual patients and their unique needs in exchange for a marketplace philosophy of lumping patients into homogenous subgroups that think and act the same; the proliferation of standardized products and services that possess mass appeal but lower levels of quality; greater potential for monopolistic delivery systems to emerge and reduce patient choice and exert disproportional influence over how parts of the system define and implement "appropriate" care; and the monetizing of doctor-patient relationships in ways that de-emphasize the cultivation of strong relational features and emphasize transactional excellence, while also pushing the notion that the doctor serves more as a "broker" helping to identify patients' needs and wants, and then connecting them with other parts of the system.

In health care, retail approaches can be used to sell an insurance plan, a specific medical service, a corporate wellness program, a new piece of office technology, or it could be used for intangible services such as convincing the patient to engage in prevention of some form, or to not seek care in a certain symptomatic situation. Regardless of the selling goal, the methods are the same—engaging consumers through multiple product or service distribution channels; using company brand to create and grow loyalty; segmenting individuals into distinct target markets; developing an efficient, customer-focused supply chain; simplifying the buying experience; creating price and quality transparency; and using analytics to buttress all of these goals (Booz and Co. 2008; Welfare 2017). The retail philosophy manifests best through a formulaic combination of interconnected strategies and tactics most effective when implemented holistically rather than as separate features. In this way, companies that do retail well embed it within every fiber of their organizational DNA. It becomes the corporate culture.

Those interested in bringing the retail philosophy to bear on the U.S. health care system generally assert that it can help to address big problems that plague the system and negatively impact cost, quality, and patient satisfaction. These problems include the lack of price and quality information on various health care products and services (e.g., How much does a knee ligament repair surgery really cost? Who is really the best surgeon to do it and why?); the lack of choice in shopping for health care products and services (e.g., my insurance plan's provider network tells me what specific doctors I can go to; my high deductible health plan makes it impossible to visit really high-quality providers because they cost more); poor alignment of patient needs and interests with existing system structures (e.g., the inability of patients to talk in real time with their physician, or immediately access their entire health record in ways that are actionable); and the complexity of a fragmented system that prevents patients from having a timely, cohesive, and simplified care-buying experience. Add to these an industry oblivious to understanding patient preferences, and there may be benefits to retail thinking in health care.

THE MAIN INGREDIENTS OF THE RETAIL PHILOSOPHY

The retail philosophy states that: (a) all those buying in a marketplace are considered "consumers"; (b) the creation and transmission of "value" to the consumer is the key way to gain competitive advantage and earn profit; (c) value is best defined by the consumer, who should be "activated" to define and seek it; and (d) establishing ongoing buyer-seller relationships that center on repeat transactions that are efficient and reliable remains the chief goal (Booz and Co. 2008). The strategies and tactics supporting this philosophy fall under two main guises: marketing and operational considerations.

Within marketing, branding and segmentation are emphasized. Branding is an organization's emphasis on establishing a specific image with the consumer that transcends any single transaction or purchase and is designed to differentiate that organization from its competitors. A company's brand is an intangible asset, one that often accounts for a large portion of its financial value as a company (Untouchable Intangibles 2014). This is because a successful brand such as Apple, Amazon, McDonald's, or Toyota by itself can guarantee a strong retail relationship between buyer and seller, and drive repeat transactions between the two parties. For example, some people will always buy Apple or Toyota products, regardless of knowing much specifically about them, because they believe in the reputation of the brand. This makes for efficient exchanges between buyer and seller, and can provide sellers with tremendous competitive advantages in the marketplace compared to others with weaker brands.

The brand reputation generally is forged over time by positive experiences between the buyer and seller (e.g., I have owned my Toyota for 10 years and I have had no major problems with it), and through the presentation of simplified metrics that convey an organization's relative positioning vis-à-vis competitors. Once a brand is strong enough, it efficiently attracts new buyers through marketing such as logos, symbols, or other devices designed to create an immediately positive perception of the organization's products in the consumer's mind. The real power of a strong brand is twofold (a) triggering a "want" and "need" in consumers, of which they may not always be fully aware; and (b) getting consumers to see these needs and wants as capable of being satisfied by a given organization.

Segmentation is the subdivision of a larger group of consumers into smaller, more homogeneous groups for the purpose of better targeting products and services, as well as better satisfying specific needs and wants (Smith 1956). Of course, given that key retail goals are *selling things* and *profit*, segmentation is intended to identify groups of consumers who present the best likelihood for both outcomes. It does not focus on the individual, but rather the group. Segmentation relies heavily on information about consumers, which gets analyzed for patterns and markers that allow aggregation. The influence of segmentation is seen in the automobile industry, where a single car brand (Toyota) has several different models marketed toward and sold to different groups of drivers. The models themselves may be differentiated according to sticker price, degree of driving luxury, environmental friendliness, size, or intent of use (e.g., pickup vs. sedan). Information on which types of drivers would buy which models is the essence of segmentation analytics. Both branding and segmentation are preoccupied with strategies and tactics involving "the 4 P's": product, price, promotion, and place.

Operational considerations in pursuing the retail philosophy focus on "value chain" management and various process improvement tools to improve the product or service workflow (Kelly 2011). These tools are preoccupied with increasing transaction speed, minimizing errors, and limiting waste. Part of this preoccupation involves the organization's general attentiveness to having economies of scale that assure good quality product or service output, and the ongoing ability to meet consumer expectations. This involves standardizing how products or services get produced and delivered wherever possible. Thus, if Amazon Prime members expect their orders to arrive reliably in the one- or two-day windows sold to them as part of their annual subscription, the company must focus operationally on creating workflows that meet this goal as close to 100 percent of the time as possible—using strategically placed fulfillment centers, tight management of product supply chains, and price competition among different package shipping companies for delivering Amazon purchases.

Technology is also at the operational heart of effective retail approaches. Retail's intense focus on repeat transactions and consumer activation lends itself to technological innovation intended primarily to move information back and forth between buyer and seller quickly; create more transparency around product price and quality; simplify and speed up the purchasing process; and position the seller in front of the buyer in as many ways as feasible. Retailers such as Amazon are successful in large part because they have used technology first and best in these ways, that is, making it easy for people to shop a range of different products online, review ratings on their relative price and quality, buy with a click of the keyboard, receive those purchases within a couple of days, and return what they wish with no questions asked. Using complex algorithms and lots of purchasing and search data, they also recommend to consumers other products that they might like to consider or buy; and use their online interface as a massive storefront where consumers can search for anything.

THE PERFECT STORM OF CIRCUMSTANCES DRIVING RETAIL INTO HEALTH CARE

Important conditions on the ground in health care provide fertile soil for growing the retail philosophy. First, many aspects of service delivery in health care remain substandard in terms of patient experience. Regarding service, health insurance plans receive some of the worst ratings in the 2016 Temkin Customer Experience Rankings (Temkin Ratings 2017). Customer experience in this survey is made up of three components—success, effort, and emotion—with success defined as the customer being able to accomplish what they set out to do; effort defined as the customer's ease of interaction with the particular company; and emotion defined as how customers felt about their specific interactions with a given company. In this survey of 10,000 consumers, the low rankings of health care plans get no better when looking at customer service and trust—two things a service industry like health care should be built upon.

Using another example of poor service and quality in health care, only 207 of 3,539 U.S. hospitals received the highest ranking of five stars from the Centers for Medicare and Medicaid Services (CMS) in their new star rating system, while a total of 714 hospitals received the lowest rankings of one or two stars (Punke 2015). The CMS rating system leans on a survey called the Hospital Consumer Assessment of Healthcare Providers and Systems (HCAHPs), which taps into a variety of patient experiences while receiving care in the hospital. It asks patients about dynamics such as communication, staff responsiveness, and other aspects of their interactions with the system. On the outpatient side, physicians and their groups also suffer poorer assessments from patients in areas such as timely access to care, providers paying attention to individuals' mental and emotional health, and providers supporting patients in taking care of their own health (Agency for Healthcare Research and Quality 2014). Besides CAHPS, there are more familiar ratings tools such as *Yelp!* that post reviews of patient experiences with doctors and hospitals. A cursory review of these ratings also suggests less than satisfactory interactions among many of us with the health care system.

Even when considering the nonclinical aspects of the health care encounter, such as a physician practice having helpful, courteous, and respectful staff, the health care industry falls short, with up to a quarter of customers in the CAHPS survey indicating that office staff do not always exhibit these characteristics. The field of primary care scores worse in all these areas compared with other specialties, perhaps because the expectations for multiple dimensions of good service and the proverbial physician bedside manner are higher. For example, in the 2014 CAHPS survey, 44 percent of the 103,000 primary care patients surveyed stated that their primary care provider did not pay attention to their mental or emotional health, two things that rely on deeper, more established doctor-patient relationships (Agency for Healthcare Research and Quality 2015). The poor service quality registered in CAHPS surveys, for example, often exists across different contexts in terms of source of care (e.g., type of practice ownership, practice size), meaning it is endemic to the entire industry.

Surveys such as CAHPS are flawed, so care must be taken in drawing firm conclusions from them. They are overly simplistic and incomplete; the questions asked often unclear or vague (e.g., "Do you like the way your provider communicated with you at your visit?" "Rate your provider from one to ten as worst possible to best possible."). The survey asks the patient not about ongoing relationships but rather a limited time span when they might have accessed care; and the questions turn most everything into a workflow or process step (Did your provider do this? Did she do that?). Tools such as *Yelp!* suffer from self-selection bias (i.e., those really happy or really angry about their experiences may tend to post reviews more frequently than others) and the posting of often highly subjective experiences, which may have less validity in the real world. Yet these tools are revealing on several different levels. First, their results help make the case for some elements of a retail approach finding their way into health care, particularly those focused on making the buying experience more satisfying. After all, how many companies successful at using retail strategies and tactics, and embedded in a highly competitive industry like health care, would tolerate a large percentage of their of their customers thinking that they did something only sporadically or not at all that was important to selling their product?

Second, survey results like these reveal inconsistencies with how individual patients think about their doctors, and perhaps the health system generally; inconsistencies that have been recognized for some time yet do inform a discussion of the doctor-patient relationship. For example, while the clinician (e.g., outpatient) version of the CAHPS survey clearly indicates that a meaningful portion of patients think their doctors (or providers as CAHPS calls them) fall short in key relational areas like communication and listening, 80 percent of them in the 2014 survey still gave their doctors a rating of 9 or 10 (out of 10) in terms of overall satisfaction (Agency for Healthcare Research and Quality 2015). This is odd to say the least.

Maybe we have some ongoing fantasy about our relationships with our doctors, or perhaps we maintain too much respect for their status, and these things undermine our willingness to lay blame directly at their doorsteps. Maybe an intimidation factor is still at work, which convinces us that if doctors do not do something needed or important for us, they must have their reasons and we should not hold it personally against them, nor expect them to try and get better. Maybe health care is one of those areas of our lives where we have gotten accustomed to poor service, accepting what is given and too afraid or ambivalent to criticize in return. If true, it raises important questions regarding our ability as consumers to hold physicians accountable, as the business owners and professionals-in-charge, for providing us with an appropriate health care delivery experience.

METRIC FEVER, CORPORATIZATION, AND THE RETAIL PHILOSOPHY

Metric fever of the kind described earlier provides the tools, data, and ways of thinking for bringing elements of retail into the health care industry. For instance, metric fever helps to facilitate: (a) simplification of the health care transaction (e.g., purchasing insurance, picking a facility or physician to go to) through more standardized, transparent indicators of quality, patient experience, and cost; and (b) patient segmentation through the use of "big data" collected through electronic health records and administrative claims databases. The heavy use of metrics also produces a steady stream of information that captures worker productivity; allows "inefficient" or "wasteful" workflows to be identified and remedied; and allows health care organizations, insurers, and patients to better understand the impact of various clinical processes on health care outcomes.

In theory, the use of metrics may promote the price competition that is a key feature of a retail-focused industry, that is, enabling sellers to undercut each other on price because they have better information to efficiently target the right kinds of customers for high-probability purchases, which, if repeated frequently, create profit margins based on transaction volume rather than high price. To understand this point, just look at what a Walmart or Amazon does, using sophisticated inventory management systems to stock lower-cost items that they know sell well, undercutting competitors on the price of those items, and then taking small profits from each item purchase that over millions of purchases add up to big profit. Metric fever in U.S. health care supports an industry-wide culture that is increasingly comfortable with "dumbing down" a variety of buyer-seller transactions, making the complex appear simple and quick. In this way, purchasing health insurance plans is done online in minutes through comparison shopping on select criteria; and patients can go onto ZocDoc and gain access to a "quality" primary care physician near them that same day.

The ongoing corporatization of primary care services is another circumstance that provides support for a growing retail approach in health care. Most importantly, this corporatization allows organizations to interact with patients more directly. As greater control is gained over key aspects of health care product or service delivery, the health care organization (e.g., hospital, physician practice, accountable care organization, insurance plan) gets chances to build its brand with patients, cultivating the latter's allegiances to it rather than to any single physician working within that organization. Thus, for example, people who live in my geographic area may consider themselves as patients of Mass General, Brigham and Women's, or Beth Israel Deaconess rather than of Dr. So and So who works for any of those systems. Thus, the organization can connect patients with the services they need or want in these systems and help them navigate the fragmentation of services that exists.

Relatedly, the corporatization of health care captures patients in ways that allow them to more easily be turned into consumers. First, as patients' reliance on a single entity for multiple types of services increases, because it is financially preferable or just plain easier, the organization or system can obtain real-time information, which allows it to know in greater depth what those patients want, need, or prefer. This reliance also establishes a greater number of "touch points" where the organization can connect with patients; provide them with positive buying experiences; and build a bond through repeat transactions. Finally, price discounts and greater "one-stop shopping" can result as the organization is able to integrate various parts of the value chain, better control upstream and downstream stakeholders (lowering the costs of production), and deliver a more seamless buying experience for the individual.

In addition, the presence of larger corporate structures such as Accountable Care Organizations (ACOs), physician super practices, and big delivery systems overseeing health care delivery means that the scale required to employ a full-bodied retail approach in health care can be met (Scheffler et al. 2016). Scale is needed for several reasons critical to retail's success: (a) the ability to engage in high-volume transactions with buyers that allow for price competition to occur and for savings to be passed onto consumers; (b) the need for a certain level of ongoing infrastructure support (e.g., technology and staffing for analytic work) to use tools such as segmentation analysis and customer experiential metrics; (c) control of multiple product distribution channels; and (d) the ability to absorb the uncertainty regarding new product or service development, subsuming financial losses for innovations that fail.

There are risks associated with pursuing the retail philosophy; risks that only larger organizations with resources can afford to take. Chief among these involves the continual innovation imperative. One need only look at the heavy financial losses retailers such as department store chains have taken in attempting to reinvent themselves in a changing marketplace to realize that bigger is better in this regard (Borchardt 2017). Health care organizations can make a case that approaching their patients through a retail lens makes sense in order to find new sources of revenue, some of which may come through nontraditional products and services, such as rewards programs and credit cards like those airlines and hotel chains offer; technological solutions that patients want; and other non-health care buying experiences. But the hard reality for these firms is that some of these products and services will hit, and others will not. An organization has to be large enough in both financial resources and market share to absorb any losses while still being able to experiment in expanding their offerings to find "the next great thing."

WORKFORCE TRANSFORMATIONS AND THE RETAIL PHILOSOPHY

Finally, the realities of various workforce transformations now occurring in the U.S. primary care system also empower the retail approach to take hold. First, as primary care physicians grow scarcer nationwide, disruptive innovations that involve more transactional exchange are introduced as outlined earlier. Driving this innovation are both health care and nonhealth care companies that already deal in retail, such as the large pharmacy chains and big-box stores. These organizations have many resources at their disposal, and see primary care as a "loss leader" providing an entrée for consumers into other areas of their business, allowing the scaling up of transactions across the product spectrum in which these consumers engage (Hoff 2013). These "innovators" tend to focus on the low-hanging fruit of easier primary care medicine, such as low-level acute care, while steering clear of care delivery that involves relational or interpersonal elements that may compete too directly with traditional primary care practices.

This approach serves their larger purpose. For example, as they open more retail clinics that can sell patients a set array of low-level primary care services cheaply because of care standardization (using clinical guidelines) and an emphasis on volume, these companies are willing to take the lower profit margins of such services in exchange for (a) building their brand with both new and existing customers (e.g., we sell you toilet paper but also take care of you when you're sick); (b) collecting information for segmentation purposes that create additional selling possibilities for related products (e.g., based on your presenting illness what prescriptions or over-the-counter products might you want to buy); and (c) introducing you to unrelated products and services in which you might have a potential interest (e.g., when you're done get 20 percent off the new smart TV on aisle 7).

Other primary care innovations involve technologies that also serve as product placement and purchasing platforms. Some of this innovation goes under the guise of "personalized health care" and includes wearable technology (e.g., fitness watches), online services such as *ZocDoc* and *ITriage*, and web-based applications involving gamification of various aspects of health care service delivery such as insurance product purchases. Although these innovations often are trumpeted in their early stages of development as revolutionary in their potential ability to engage people in their health care, improve care quality, and improve convenience in accessing care, there is little current systematic evidence they achieve any of these outcomes in meaningful ways right now.

Discussed less often is how the companies driving such innovation, many from outside of health care, such as *Apple* or *Nike*, see their products as a means to extend existing brand strength and loyalty into the health care area; create consumer demand in untapped niche areas where quick market share and profits can be had (i.e., the type of low-hanging fruit mentioned above); and advertise other health and non-health related products sold by themselves and third-party vendors, gaining revenue in the process. In these ways, the workforce changes occurring that involve fewer primary care physicians; greater use of health care teams; and the upskilling of semiskilled health workers to perform more complex work open the door for new ideas about how to think about and provide primary care—new ideas that are generated mainly by retail-focused companies often looking to sell more things to people, rather than by the medical profession.

Relatedly, the innovations touted as enhancements to primary care delivery also serve to embed and spread the retail philosophy among health care customers in other covert ways. For example, the fitness watch or smartphone app that gathers your health-related data in real-time may sell the information collected to others or use it directly to advertise specific products and services to you, ones that you may or may not need. One 2013 study showed that the 20 most frequently used fitness apps passed consumer information they collected along to almost 70 other companies (Harding 2013). In this and similar ways, such technology is also designed to get you connected to other possible economic transactions offered up by companies not associated with the original health care innovation.

Workforce transformations that involve the development of new or enhanced skill sets among a variety of health care occupations such as nursing and medical assisting also feed into growth of the retail philosophy. First, relying on non-physician labor that is lower paid and more controllable allows health care organizations to experiment with retail-focused ideas in the workplace in an efficient manner, with less resistance from the worker (e.g., physician) side. In addition, compared to training more doctors, semiskilled support occupations like medical assisting can be built up relatively quickly in terms of numbers (Bureau of Labor Statistics 2017) to interact directly with patients across a variety of care issues and areas. Focusing more on these semiskilled occupations to support the organization-customer interface takes consumer engagement tactics somewhat out of the physician's hands. These support workers provide the organization with greater ability to connect with patients, versus working through physicians or even nurses whose professional identification may subvert their interests in representing the organization to the customer.

VOICES FROM THE TRENCHES: EXPLORING HOW DOCTORS AND PATIENTS EXPERIENCE THEIR RELATIONSHIPS

The remainder of the book, with the exception of the final chapter, lets primary care doctors and patients weigh in on how their relationship looks right now, how it is changing, and whether it is conceived and enacted in the spirit of loftier traditional ideals, harsher contextual realities, or some combination of both. It examines how these two parties make sense of their interactions with each other; what their experiences with each other are now like; and what their expectations are of the relationship itself. This book is novel in that I do not think such topics previously have been explored systematically or in-depth. Each of the three data chapters that follow present findings around various themes that emerge from my interviews with doctors and patients, and then critically analyze the implications of those themes for the future of the doctor-patient relationship, the retail philosophy, and the future personality of the health care industry itself. Part of the examination also seeks to understand the rivals for patient attention in the relational sphere, such as the health care organization, and whether those rivals are making inroads into the hearts and minds of patients. In the final analysis, it is the *lived experience* of the doctor-patient relationship that matters. So some of that experience is described and analyzed here. It can inform some of the issues raised in these first three chapters.

One issue is the marked contrast between the retail philosophy and its emphasis on the organization (seller)–customer (buyer) relationship, and the dyadic doctor-patient relationship, which, at its best, involves strong interpersonal bonds between professional and client. The voices present here, though small in number, represent some of the first to help us understand if the reified image of the doctor-patient relationship fits the reality before us, and if both doctor and patient want that reified image, or something else. A second issue that the voices in this book speak to is how much the various contextual issues described in the prior pages are impacting the potential for fully functioning doctor-patient relationships in primary care. What sort of workplace and interactional environments now exist for doctors and patients to even consider acting toward each other in a highly relational manner? Or is the retail philosophy and some of its ideas better aligned with the everyday reality of where U.S. health care delivery is going?

Despite the lead-up of these first chapters, and their somewhat critical tone, no firm conclusions have been drawn ahead of time regarding, for example, how both doctors and their patients feel about or experience their relationship today. No particular innovation is thrown under the bus; no single stakeholder is identified as the prime suspect; and no specific ideology is cast as either complete hero or villain. Rather, the cold calculus of reality as it pertains to the world doctors and their patients now find themselves within—some of it thrust upon them and some of it created by their own hand—is illuminated. It is a world with its share of key ironies, wishful thinking, frustrated and confused people, and deeply moving interpersonal experiences. That said, it is also a world that clearly has changed, that continues to evolve rapidly, and one in which the physician may soon give way to the health care organization as the central figure for patients, not only in primary care but across the entire spectrum of health care delivery. The final chapter attempts not to avoid the realities articulated in Chapters 4 through 6, but instead to offer up several strategic responses that might preserve a healthy dose of relational care between doctor and patient within the system at all times; raise the expectations for that care among doctors and patients; and give health care organizations and the retail philosophy a reason for paying attention to it. The next chapter gives us a glimpse into how doctors see their relationships with patients.

Chapter 4

All Roads Lead to Trust

*How Doctors See the Relationship
and Our Expectations*

In interviews, physicians seemed to romanticize the doctor-patient relationship. Like the literature discussed in Chapter 1, the doctors interviewed in this study talked in very personal and idealistic terms about the softer qualities that they believed went into a strong, effective, and satisfying union between doctor and patient. They emphasized the positive feelings and good medicine that resulted from having patients with whom they could establish connections on both emotional and psychological levels. Their vision of the best relationships were focused less directly on doing *the right things clinically* and instead on creating *relational states with patients* that enhanced trust. These relational states were hard to standardize, took time, depended on a great deal of situational behavior and serendipity, and did not easily fit into a set of metrics. Overall, doctors discussed their best relationships with patients in ways that focused on the best of what each party could experience when given a chance to interact directly with one another over time. From my own perspective as a patient, listening to these physicians talk in this way was both refreshing and seductive. In key ways, however, it also seemed misaligned with the larger realities of health care delivery today and the retail approach slowly being embraced by health care organizations.

Contextually, time and ongoing contact were important factors in forging strong relationships. In addition, all physicians portrayed the doctor-patient relationship as one that by definition involved a mix of situational paternalism and coequality, both dynamics acting on a foundation of belief that each of the two stakeholders would know how this particular mix should play out in a given care instance. This was one of the big challenges identified. From the doctor's perspective, simultaneously acting as an authoritative professional figure *and* a trusted confidante was the most complex aspect of the job to pull off in the course of relating to a given patient over time.

> I think that they [my patients] see the relationship as really unique where I am someone that can in some sense, be treated like a friend. They open up to me. They talk to me as they would their friend, but in another sense I have that other level where I have to give guidance and things like that. (Rachel)

> There are two things that have to exist simultaneously. You have to have boundaries with those folks, emotional boundaries. You can be supportive and be a good listener, but they need to know that there are certain things you can and can't do, certain things you have to do for them. (Pete)

In the best of circumstances, what starts out for the primary care physician as an unknown patient waiting in the exam room becomes more through years of periodic yet steady direct contact. It blossoms into a faithful, mutually beneficial association that allows many other necessary things to be attempted and done in terms of diagnosis and treatment. One young physician touched on this point when describing a seminal moment in her own training, when she was on one of her clinical rotations:

> I remember one patient that was seeing the doctor I was with, who was coming in every month and was pretty depressed. And you could feel the palpable relief in the room when she [the patient] was in there with him [the doctor] because he knew her, he knew her situation. I felt like she was able to trust him, and they were able to really work on a continuing plan for her depression because they had already had that relationship. With something

like mental illness, that kind of thing can really make or break the treatment. That patient really stood out to me and got me thinking more about what a relationship with my patients could be like. As opposed to other experiences in my rotations where I saw someone in the hospital, and they got a diagnosis and then I never saw them again. (Olivia)

The best relationships in this regard were not cited by the physicians interviewed as occurring for all of their patients. In fact, one of the hard-to-figure aspects of these discussions with doctors was trying to determine when someone was talking from a deep, rich reservoir of actual experience and when they were drawing more on a limited example supplemented by their own imagination or wishful thinking to produce a desired vision of an effective relationship. Even when asked about it directly, most doctors could not quantify the extent to which in their careers they had been a part of the ideal-type relationships they described. This was where the more romanticized feeling came into play: I was often unsure if some physicians were asserting these relational qualities to help convince themselves of the way things should be, rather than are, in the midst of an everyday world revolutionizing around them.

Some doctors, particularly older ones, talked about having many such relationships, and they described some of them in-depth. Other doctors were less specific, and at times talked about the best patient relationships in more elusive terms. In any event, few physicians flinched when asked to describe what they felt a good doctor-patient relationship looked like, despite some having extensive firsthand knowledge and others knowing it more distally. Everyone had stories illuminating their perceptions of a strong doctor-patient relationship. There was a consistent drumbeat across interviews in the types of relational features most emphasized as important, and why. Striking to me was the consistent manner in which doctors specifically used the words trust, respect, friendship, partnership, and communication to help describe an effective, satisfying doctor-patient relationship. They used these words unprompted, and in purposeful ways meant to convey how important social interaction with patients was in their work.

MASTERING THE HUMAN ELEMENT
IN PATIENT CARE

For the physicians interviewed, it was not being good diagnostic technicians, chronic disease managers, care coordinators, metric masters, or
"value-enhancing" clinicians that in their experiences or eyes made them
good doctors or produced meaningful connections with patients. They
felt that these work roles were the preoccupation of the organizations and
insurance companies with whom they dealt. They talked about fulfilling
these roles as strategic necessities thrust onto them to get paid or maintain
good relationships with insurance plans or employers, rather than with
patients. In this regard, some of the interviewees came across as prison-
ers of their existing work circumstances. And whether true or not, they
also believed to a person that patients cared much less about these other
roles, most of which for doctors could not meet the full range of a patient's
needs, or cater to the patient as a unique human being. Physicians thought
that being a good manager of chronic diseases in patients, for example, or
a sound technician in terms of knowing how to fulfill the requirements of
a quality checklist for a given patient, was something that had its place,
but not in helping to establish strong emotional and psychological bonds
between doctor and patient, or in ultimately providing the best care
possible.

> I would make the argument that any given individual is more
> than a collection of their metrics. You and I could look identical
> on paper and be radically different, for example, that you calling
> me up and saying you have chest pain and I calling you up and
> saying I have chest pain are radically different experiences. There
> are patients, and I got one just the other day, the guy came in
> and he looked fine on paper. His numbers were fine. But he said
> to me, "I just feel terrible." And so I knew something was wrong.
> Because this is a guy I've known for 15 years; he's never said he
> feels terrible. His leg could be chopped off but he would still say
> he's fine. So if you don't know the guy, you might not take him
> seriously. (Hal)

Some people feel it's [focus on guideline compliance] just the way the business is now and we just have to try to do what we can. I think it's – they'll make the case: Well, it's getting more of the right things done and you can't deny that and so you can't fight with it. You know I do a micro albumin test on someone who you know has already moderate renal insufficiency and is already on maximal therapy for what you treat the albuminuria for, and you do the test not because it's really going to help the person any but because you need that number so you can fill it into the blank, OK, all right? I mean it's not harmful to the patient but is it going to change anything? I helped them? Absolutely not, OK? (Curt)

It's interesting because my intuition and bias has always been that there's a lot of value to really having that relationship and knowing your patient. The other side of the argument is that really the key aspect of quality is more the ability to follow a checklist and well-established guidelines. If you actually do all these things regardless of whether you know the patient from Adam, will you have better outcomes? At least my own instinct is that in the primary care setting the relationship is paramount and perhaps if you're in an ICU setting, conforming to a checklist might be more relevant at least in the immediate sense. A patient there could pretty well accept that you do things by the book every time. (Billy)

Their own ability to *relate* to patients on deeper psychological and emotional levels was the key focus for them in their work. They emphasized this point at every turn. This meant proving to the patient not that they knew when and how to push for a specific type of screening or lab test to be done, for example, but instead that they could listen and learn, be trusted, provide emotional support, keep things in confidence, and give expert advice but not dictate. It also meant knowing important things about a patient's life story; knowing when to probe deeper into a patient's condition; when appropriate, showing the patient some degree of professional vulnerability in terms of having clinical doubts; and connecting with each individual in ways that made them feel the physician was a real person, in key ways just like them.

Certainly, fulfilling additional work roles, for example as care coordinator, helped doctors to bond with their patients, providing reliable experiences (if done well) that increased confidence in the doctor's competence. But these other work roles were not the major drivers of trust in the relationship. For doctors, relating in a complex, multifaceted way that emphasized softer interpersonal attributes was neither easy nor quick. It depended on tacit agreements between doctor and patient that created a dual sense of emotional accountability, which for the physician was facilitated by adequate time together, timely access, and frequent direct contact.

> Well, it takes time to get to know someone. The whole thing is built on trust, but trust takes some time. For example, I would talk to a patient who I've known for four years differently than I talk to someone who I've known for two months. I think to build trust, you really have to show that you're gonna be there. You're willing to meet them where they're at. You're not judging them. You're in it to help them. It's kind of like being a parent in some cases where a kid might come to you finally when they're ready to talk. It's the same with a patient. Time is important. You need to provide enough time in the room. Access is important. Patients need to feel like they can talk to you or get to you, that there's not major barriers to care in terms of access. (Pete)

Some doctors highlighted how different their experiences were with patients with whom no mutual trust or sense of connection yet existed.

> There's a heightened level of anxiety for me going into the rooms of patients that I don't know. Partially because I know that they don't know me, and they may not trust me. Also, I just don't know or trust them. I can look at their chart, I can look at their problem list, but it doesn't tell me everything that is going on. It doesn't mean I know them. And I hear the patient's frustration of having to repeat their story to somebody new every time. So, I go in there wanting to do right by them, but I know I can't figure it all out in one visit. The twenty minutes I have isn't going to be enough. Whereas with my

existing patients that I know well, that twenty minutes plays out very differently. (Olivia)

Given that doctors emphasized the human elements, the best relationships came across as more organic and situational, forged through extended social interactions that allowed for serendipity in what doctors could discover about their patients. Organic in the sense of having relational features able to occur naturally. Situational in terms of how the particular doctor and patient involved might shape these human elements, and also how other aspects of the surrounding context (e.g., time, the patient's condition) affected the extent to which such elements could manifest. Doctors talked about their best patient relationships in ways that conveyed a high comfort level with the uncertainty associated with implementing features such as empathy and listening. But when they felt they did not know a patient well enough, or did not believe in the relationship as a whole yet, they were subject to greater apprehension and unease in how they went about their work, and they held back.

ALL ROADS LEAD TO TRUST

The word "trust" came out of physicians' mouths more than any other when defining a strong, satisfying doctor-patient relationship. Trust was identified as the social glue giving their patient relationships staying power. In particular, the willingness for patients to confide in their doctor, to express vulnerability, to allow the physician to take action, to want to come back, and to believe that the physician would try his best to advise and behave in the patient's best interests—these were the benefits of relational trust. In many ways, how these doctors discussed trust and its implications for their work was consistent with how the literature has portrayed the concept, discussed in Chapter 1. They valued it above all else.

I only have my perceptions about my patients' perceptions and what I get out of the relationship most importantly is the concept of being trusted. I find that very rewarding. (Keith)

As noted in Chapter 1, trust involves one party's willingness to be vulnerable to another's behavior with the expectation that the former will benefit from that behavior (Mayer et al. 1995). This definition came out in how doctors talked about the term:

> I think the basic thing is trust. They have to have faith that I know what I'm doing and that I care about them and that I'm going to follow through on what I say. I think that's the main thing, you know in order to establish that, obviously you have to see the patient. You have to have enough contacts with them that they kind of know who you are and you know who they are and you have established some sort of rapport. (Betsey)

The type of trust discussed was exclusively *relational* in nature. For example, none of the physicians referred to the instrumental forms of trust that increasingly were pushed onto them through linking their pay to the performance of certain work tasks (e.g., chronic disease management, care coordination) and clinical processes (e.g., recommending colorectal screening for all patients over 50 years of age) meant on paper to benefit the patient. In fact, none of the physicians interviewed ever suggested that their desired form of trust was the kind that involved making sure "things were done" in a manner consistent with a written clinical guideline or Patient-Centered Medical Home checklist. There was a notable absence of focus on the more easily measurable work processes as sources for developing lasting bonds with patients. Rather, these physicians emphasized the interpersonal side of their work when articulating to me the development and use of trust to deliver good medicine. Consider the following anecdotes from doctors' work experiences:

> One of my patients came to me one day, we were doing a fair amount of OB and she said, you know, this is my third pregnancy. She said my last pregnancy, my labor lasted 20 minutes and I live in [Town A], and [Town A] is 15 minutes from my office and another 15 minutes from the hospital. I was kind of mid-way but I said let's do this. If you get into labor I said I'll meet you down at the office,

I'll deliver you there. I mean I don't think you're gonna make it. I said if you're gonna deliver, you can deliver it anywhere. I mean people deliver in cabs. I said at least I'll have it an appropriate delivery tray so that we could just deliver the baby, no problem. Well back then, we did a lot of work in ICUs and CCUs, and I happened to have been on call up in the hospital, and I was in the intensive care unit and she called me and she said *I'm in labor* and I said well, you know, here's the deal, have your husband get you into the truck and bring you up here because I can't meet you down at the office. So about half an hour later I get a call from the emergency room. He said you'd better get down here, your patient's out in the parking lot and it was first part of December. So I ran down, I grabbed the nurse and delivered her on the front seat of her husband's truck. I carried the baby over after I cut the cord, carried the baby over into the emergency room. The steam is rising off of the kid. That's what I remember because obviously the kid's 98.6 degrees and he's covered with amniotic fluid but the kicker to the whole thing was she had ruptured her membranes in the front seat of her husband's truck, and of course you know what a mess that is. The guy had the old-fashioned plastic seat covers all over the seats. So I could imagine he just went home and took a hose, and just hosed down the front of the car. (Owen)

A lot of my younger patients have depression and anxiety, and they don't want to see a psychiatrist, either they don't have time or there's a stigma or the psychiatrist wants to prescribe medicine. I'm certainly not a therapist. I don't pretend to be, but I think a lot of patients treat me in that respect where they just kind of want to have someone to bounce ideas off of or talk about issues. I've had a lot of patients, they'll do this like, "Oh, do you think I should break up with my boyfriend? Oh, do you think I should do this?" I'm like, "I can't make that decision for you," but I try to at least help them come to their own conclusion, I guess, and stuff. (Ola)

I have a patient that we found had a renal mass during hospitalization in the spring. And I referred her to the urologist here and our chest surgeon 'cause she had pulmonary nodules. And so we were gonna work through it. And her family said, "Oh no, no, we're gonna take her to Sloan-Kettering." And so through the summer I would get things from them saying that she saw this specialist and she needed that MRI but couldn't do it and they were driving back and forth. Finally in September they came to me in crisis, mom won't go back to New York City and she just wants to die and it took three visits to kind of sort through what was happening. Part of it was she didn't want to be going down there. It was really hard. They thought they were doing the right thing for her but they weren't listening to what she felt she needed and they weren't getting any communication from the specialist. They were seeing the specialist from Kettering, a guy that does the left renal masses and when she said, "I have pain on the right side," he said, "Well it's not your kidney." You know and that was the end of the discussion with him on her pain on the right side that happened to be on the other side from where her mass was. Working with that family was good for me. I mean, it made me feel good that I could help them negotiate through that. (Betsey)

You know the person; you know the family; oftentimes, you know multiple members of the family. It's very personal, and especially for some of the more complicated patients. I had a patient, for example, who had multiple chronic medical problems. She actually followed me to [Town B], and she just passed away about two months ago. I had taken care of all her family. She would basically rely upon me to try and help interpret a lot of the stuff that was going on with her other specialists. She had a cardiologist, and she had a GI doctor, and she had a pulmonologist. She had multiple systems failure. And by keeping that together and also staying in touch with the doctors, I felt that I was able to, number one, keep her really large medication list under some level of control and be able to actually triage her issues prior to them getting more severe. That was part of it. Part of it was the fact that she was also really chronically ill, and so I was just a touchstone. I couldn't fix everything, but she could basically come in, tell me what was going on, and I could sort of give her a sense as to what might be more serious, what needed further evaluation, and what was really something that was part of her chronic situation that we were just going to sort of watch and see where it goes. I think that, in that sense, the fact that I'd known her for 20 years and taken care of her for 20 years, through multiple illnesses, including hospitalizations—there was an ability to actually sort of assess and reassure, where there was some element of reassurance, and get her into more advanced care when that needed to be done. She was the kind of person who was always sort of on the abyss, in terms of her health. And I felt that, for the many years I knew her, I was able to sort of play that role. She and her mother, who I had cared for—and her niece, who I cared for—sort of would rely upon me for that, as well. So, they might go and see all the other doctors, but at the same time, I was sort of—I was kind of almost an interpreter of what was going on with all the other folks. (Bobby)

I went into the grocery store probably a month ago and before I had left I had bumped into three different people; two of which were having family problems. One was a husband and one was a grand-son, and right in the middle of the supermarket I get into a discussion and they break down in tears. Everybody is walking around, is wondering what the hell is going on, and they still feel that they can stop me no matter where I am and just kind of say can you help me out here and can you lend an ear. (Billy)

You know there's something called a thoracentesis. That's where you put a needle into somebody's chest to remove fluid or to remove air. I had a lady who was a very good friend of mine, actually a mother of a schoolmate of my older brother's, and she had lung cancer and she wanted to die at home and she didn't want to go in the hospital. And three times a week I would finish up at the office and actually do something that nobody else would do and that is I would drive over to her house which was on the way to my home, and I would put a needle into her back right there in her house and drain off as much fluid as I needed to so that she could breathe before she ultimately died in her sleep. It just gave her the time that she needed to spend with her husband and at a level of comfort before she peacefully met the maker. (Owen)

As the anecdotes imply and physicians emphasized, trust specifically enabled them to take greater risks in doing things for patients. It motivated them to be more involved in their patients' lives, to try and understand them better as unique individuals instead of aggregate groups of diseases or symptoms. In one instance, it enabled a parking lot delivery. In another, it encouraged them to move past the overt complaint and immediate service need, and into doing something more focused on the patient's underlying problems. In a third, it made the physician self-confident enough to give over care of his patients to others while still feeling responsible for them. Overall, it pushed all of them to a higher level of engagement in their patients' situations.

> There are some things that you need to think more broadly about. Trust helps. A patient can be complex for a lot of reasons, not just diagnosis. The alcoholic comes in with a laceration. Took care of the laceration, but did you help them with their problem? Who's gonna do that? That kind of care. And there are a lot of folks like this, the depressed person who you know keeps coming back for that stomach pain. You're going to spend a lot of time and money. Keep coming back. How many CT scans are you gonna do, and how long is it gonna take before you realize that there might be more going on that meets the eye. Maybe they're getting the shit beaten out of them at home. Did you ask them? And even if you did ask them, then what are you doing about it? (Liza)

From the doctor's perspective, trust also moved the relationship toward a true professional-client partnership whereby a common set of understandings could be reached about the patient's condition, and this enhanced care in their eyes. For the primary care physician especially, the cultivation of this type of partnership had practical implications, such as patients staying with them longer in a given care situation versus being referred out to other parts of the system to receive services.

> Guy comes in—a veteran who's been bopping in and out of shelters, bopping in and out of the VA, happened to be stumbling in this area, there wasn't a VA here. He's like, "Doc, I can't see that great." The dude had diabetes, raging diabetes. That's why he couldn't see

great, 'cause his sugar was so high it was affecting his vision. He was thrilled to get a diagnosis, which you could say anyone could do. But what he did next was rare. So he's a guy bopping around, doesn't have any relationship with anybody in the system. But he started to come in, he wanted to know what he could do. I helped coordinate how to get him to an eye doc, 'cause he was already starting to have some retinopathy, got him education on his diabetes, and I helped direct other providers and did follow-up visits with him, asking him how he felt. And he responded, telling me that "when I ate this thing doc, my sugars went way up, and when I take this medicine it goes up, but not as much." It all helped him understand what I was getting at. So then he was more bought into stuff, and he was feeling better. So he kept coming back, which was awesome. And we helped his numbers get so much better, like an A1C from a 12 down to the realm of sevens, really shockingly low. (Liza)

Some patients really have a little higher level of trust and therefore aren't wanting to be quick to go out to specialty care, whereas other patients are very quick to want to see a specialist for this or that very, very quickly. I think that's mostly due to patients' perception. I think patients more and more perceive that sometimes specialty care is better. Maybe they don't have a basic trust in the primary care doctor. But I think for the doctor themselves, I think most of us take our cues as to how quickly to refer or quickly to maintain patients, we take it from what the patient urges us, or pushes us, or wants us to do. That's the way I kind of look at it. (Bradley)

FRIENDS AND ADVISORS: DUAL ROLES NEEDED TO BECOME A TRUSTED PHYSICIAN

A necessary relational element that was a building block of the trust required for a strong, effective, and satisfying doctor-patient relationship involved physicians fulfilling two roles simultaneously with a patient, namely that of friend *and* expert advisor. These roles blended for doctors such that it was unclear as they discussed them where one fully ended and another began. Friendship played out a little differently across physicians, depending upon where they practiced geographically and how long they had been in practice. But the overall meaning of friendship for these doctors was based in a sense of recognition by their patients that there was someone they were seeing with whom they could identify.

> I wouldn't say that my patients are my personal friends; you know we're not hanging out on the weekend barbecuing, but these are people clearly with whom I have a personal relationship. (Hal)

> You don't want to be best friends with your patients, but you need them to know that you're a human being, that they're talking to another human being. (Scott)

At a macro level, such feelings of friendship on the physician's part fed into a stronger sense that they (the physician) were tied into the community in which they worked, accepted by those who lived around them, and recognized simultaneously as both a subject matter expert and close confidante. Physicians seemed to derive a strong sense of their work identity and career satisfaction from this realization.

> The physician in my day, you know, was part of the family. I didn't have a beeper but people knew my number at home and they didn't mind calling me. If you went to a function some people would just pull you aside and say, you know, I've got this kind of a problem. Do you think—can we talk about it here or do you think I ought to come in and see you? But it's that sense and a lot of the doctors, when I was in private practice, they were part of the community. I think that that's a real important aspect of the provision of health care. I think that you have to become part of the community in order to understand first of all some of the things that you wouldn't, if you kind of went to work in the morning and came home, and were a part of the elite. You've got to understand that you've gotta be down to earth about this and you can't hold your head too high. (Owen)

I'm in a small rural community that is kind of connected to a critical access hospital. So with that, we're really maybe one of two or three primary care physicians in the area within a 30-mile radius. The patient population that I get to see is really familiar to me. I know great grandma, grandpa, dad, baby, four generations of patients, sprinkled in with their dogs and cats and horses, and everything in between. So you really feel like you are part of the family, you get invited to baptisms and birthday parties and it's just a very close feeling. (Uma)

In the vast literature on professionals that exists, both conceptual and empirical, the notion that elite workers such as doctors seek or need to maintain psychological and emotional distance from their clients is taken as a given (Larson 1977; Spangler 1986; Starr 1982). The rationale for this assumption lies in the notion that through this distance, a professional's expertise is applied more objectively to a client's situation, removing potential conflicts of interest and variability in service delivery that derive from the doctors' own internal biases from knowing the patient too well. It would remove the potential for quackery that was tied to a professional performing work and making decisions based more in what they believed the client wanted (e.g., to satisfy them and make them want to use the professional again) rather than in good evidence or science. As a sociologist, I learned early in my studies that experts such as physicians and lawyers also gained some of their cultural legitimacy with the public by promoting a sense that their training and experiences gave them a superior point of view on the needs of their clients; one not to be overly questioned by the latter. Yet, to almost all of the doctors interviewed, what they saw as their best relationships were the ones in which they felt a sense of *commonality* with the patient.

In their experience, establishing this type of rapport facilitated interpersonal trust between doctor and patient on several levels. First, it made patients more willing to be honest with the physician, and perhaps share things that they (the patients) were confused or uncomfortable about revealing. This enhanced the likelihood that physicians would make better, timelier diagnoses in areas such as mental health, where symptoms might be masked or misinterpreted given their hidden nature. In this way, developing friendship-type bonds with some patients was a crucial element in gaining insight into a patient's "subterranean" needs, that is, those issues and needs that were not directly observable, not easily captured through application of a guideline or test, and often not fully known by patients' themselves.

Second, this rapport helped the physicians share with patients some of their own feelings of vulnerability in relation to their work, which they (the physicians) saw as important for getting patients to place their faith in them. This was a somewhat counterintuitive notion. That is, for physicians, it was not appearing infallible or robotically efficient in the application of their medical knowledge that made patients trust them. Rather, it was having the patient know that his doctor was a flesh-and-blood human being like him, not all-knowing or perfect, but instead an expert who had limitations in the scope of her knowledge, someone who made mistakes, and someone who could not predict or see all that was going on.

> The other piece of that is to be consistent in letting them know where your limitations are in knowledge, so if I don't know how to treat their—if their toe gets big and red being able to say, "Well, you know, I'm not exactly sure what to do here, but we'll get you to somebody that can help." (Karen)

> I think first of all most of my patients were friends. They came to me because, number one, they felt that they could talk to me. Number two, they felt that I was capable enough to take care of their problems and, number three, they felt that I was capable enough, if I couldn't take care of their problems I could get them to somebody who could. (Owen)

Of course, this perception might have been more typically found within primary versus specialty care. Patients view specialists as technicians (as we will see) who need to get things right, given that their role is a narrower one, that is, to fix a specific problem already identified as requiring intervention. Bedside manner is less important than good technique in the application of corrective measures such as surgery. Although physicians valued the emotional and practical aspects of feelings of friendship with their patients, and believed this helped create trust within the relationship, this was not friendship in the most ordinary sense, because along with it came the role of physicians being the experts who were required by their licensure, training, and a set of patient expectations to provide formal guidance about their patients' care. During interviews, most doctors emphasized, sometimes in the very next sentence after discussing "patient friendships," their need to serve in this other expert role. This role was more emotionally detached and heavily rooted in application of the physician's diagnostic skills and medical knowledge.

> Patients are coming to you as an expert and they're looking for at the very least an opinion on something that they don't know or else they wouldn't come in most of the time. (Dana)

> I usually tell people it's like this. When I go to my mechanic, he's the expert. I trust his opinion, and I do want him to tell me what to do because I don't have any idea, especially with new, modern cars that are so computerized. I don't know what's going on under the hood anymore. I do want him to tell me what to do. I think that it's not necessarily a bad thing when we as physicians tell patients, "This is really the best thing. As a team, we can decide together what the approach to that end should be, but I really do think this is the best thing for you." And relying on physicians as the expert again, because I think we got away from that in the politically correct thinking and, "Oh, paternalistic medicine is bad." Well, I don't think it's bad, I just think that maybe we need to refocus it. (Harry)

Being an expert advisor involved a range of behaviors from providing counsel to patients, allowing the latter to ultimately decide if and how to use such counsel, to acting in a more directive role and getting patients to take a decisive action, put forth by the physician, with respect to their health care. Consistent with the overall theme emerging from discussions with physicians, little of the expert advisor role was couched in a focus on getting patients to comply with standardized guidelines, although it was entirely possible physicians avoided telling me that such a focus was part of this role because of their own feelings of negativity around checklist care. However, I sensed on their part a vaguely construed everyday enactment of this expert advisor role, that is, it came across as such an engrained component of their interactions with patients that it was enacted in less prescribed ways by the physician.

LISTEN AND LEARN: HEARING
THE PATIENT'S STORY

Perhaps the most talked about aspect of building trust with patients was the need to be a good listener and, more importantly, to use one's listening ability as a means to get to know patients, identify their most important care needs, and figure out the best ways to interact with them as unique individuals. These physicians placed a lot of faith in the listening aspect of their jobs, and believed that pragmatically it helped them achieve greater patient compliance as well as trust with their patients.

> I really think it's just listening to the patient. It's really amazing if you just don't say anything and let them talk for a good amount of time. It's surprising what people will bring up to you. (Rachel)

> I have a patient that was new to me here when I got here. She'd been here before. In the first visit, I really kind of just. . . I forget what I even asked up front but I let her talk for a good—I don't know how long it was, but it seemed like a long time and she felt it was a long time, 'cause then I did at some point say, "OK, let's go back to whatever," and at the end of that visit, she deliberately said, "I felt like you really listened to me in the beginning. You didn't cut me off with it." So since then, we've actually been able to make medication adjustments and she agrees with them. We talked about recommendations for things and she goes like, "OK. I trust you." And I think that really started with literally the first five minutes of letting her talk." (Dana)

As in the discussion of feelings of friendship, emphasizing the listening aspect of their jobs facilitated physicians' ability to deliver "subterranean care." To hear these physicians tell it, many patients came into the primary care setting with immediate needs and overt symptoms that often lay at the tip of a proverbial iceberg of deeper, less well understood problems, which might or might not reveal themselves in the course of a face-to-face visit, or anyplace else in their encounters with the health care system. For these doctors, true prevention and good medicine was not simply reacting to what a prescribed guideline or checklist called for or what the initial presentation of symptoms implied, but also looking for signs of other maladies and, equally important, trying to identify clues in the patient's body language and own words that suggested the need for additional touch points and inquiry. In their experience, not only did engaging in active listening allow physicians to improve the chances patients might, either purposefully or serendipitously, come to bond in a more intimate way with them, it also helped physicians cultivate interpersonal features such as empathy and respect that made them better clinicians.

You can't be judgmental. You just listen. These folks with anxiety, depression, or worse mental illness, they have a tough life typically. They have strained relationships. Often they felt like they have disclosed it to another provider, whether it's a doctor or a counselor, who kind of blew them off. I think patient education goes a long way and also just listening, just bearing witness and giving them some hope that things can get better. Convince them that this is a place where you're safe, and you can come, and we'll listen to you, and we're gonna try to help you. You move slowly. Unless their life is in danger or someone else is in danger, you move very slowly. Often those people have other issues, either alcoholism or they're in for headaches or stomach aches or pain everywhere. You can really couch it to them as, "People have different responses to stress, and your body's response might be that you get headaches or that you drink a little too much to help you feel better," and try to get rid of any of the stigma that goes along with it, especially in guys, the 60-year-old guys and blue-collar guys who don't want to talk about this stuff. I think you really have to package it—make it a very physical thing, because in their mind it's weakness. There's something wrong with them. They're just weak. They just need to tough it out and get over it. So it's time. It's listening. It's telling them, "You've got these headaches. Let's just try doing—let's try—humor me." Sometimes I'll say, "Just humor me and try this medication and see if it helps you. Then come back and see me in two weeks." Then they see you in two weeks, and you say, "Come back and see me in two weeks again." And usually by the third or fourth visit they are ready to talk about what's really bothering them. (Pete)

A gentleman, in his late fifties, who had had a serious heart attack a few years prior, came in to see me, and he was not much engaged in his own care. I had this agenda in my head of the things I was going to talk to him about, and the third time he came in he just started crying, talking about how he had been feeling really depressed, how he'd been the guy who worked all his life, and—you know, he wasn't able to do that anymore, and not able to provide and he just felt like a failure. And getting past that, I mean was huge. (Barbara)

Listening was an important activity with many benefits for physicians and their relationships with patients. In short, it was a crucial part of their professional toolbox, that is, another relational feature that made them feel as though they were really helping their patients.

So you have to not just listen, but also help kind of, you know, figure out what really matters to the patient. They want to feel heard but there's also a thing that they care about. They'll tell the doctor it if the doctor keeps listening, and that brings it all together. (Bridget)

I think when you get the chance to talk to the patient, and you get that, "Oh, is that the injury you were talking about that you had when you were 12?" That part makes you feel like a physician, I think, and putting it together and piecing it together and being like, "OK, this is what I think it is." And having that relationship with your patient and being able to say, "I'm not sure, but I think it's either this, this, or this." I feel like that takes so much burden off of the patient and they feel like, even if you didn't do anything, "OK, somebody's thinking about my problem, somebody wants to treat my problem, and this is our plan for going through that." (Cleo)

I had a younger patient, a teenager, whom I had seen several times before. And he came in for a visit, and he just wasn't right, he was flat, and so I asked his mother to leave the room and I went through all the questions, was he taking any drugs, the standard things. And at the very end of all that I asked "Is there anything else you want to talk about before your Mom comes back in?" And he said "I don't have feelings anymore. I used to be happy and I want to be happy again." He kept talking, and he said he hadn't told anyone how he was feeling, not his Mom, no one. So he asked for help, and coming from a younger boy, that's huge. I felt like I made it comfortable for him to talk. (Olivia)

ACCOUNTABILITY: LETTING PATIENTS KNOW YOU'RE THERE FOR THEM

For physicians, trust could not occur without accountability, and an effective doctor-patient relationship required it. Accountability for them was defined chiefly as (a) being accessible to patients in a timely manner, and (b) once accessible, providing patients with adequate contact time, be it through face time or virtual communications.

You know I think being available is important because if you're not there when things happen then you know, you don't form those bonds that you would form otherwise. So when our office is closed one of us is taking phone calls. And the beauty of it is that our patients don't abuse that. It's very rare that I get a call from somebody for something that could've been done during office hours. So I think that's helpful because you know again it lets them know that you're there and that you care. (Betsey)

You have this doctor-patient relationship that is really sacrosanct and you have to value that and own it. When someone's sick you should be available. You should take responsibility. It's very difficult to step back from that a little bit and say there's going to be a co-ownership or you're going to delegate it to someone else. (Billy)

We can all run reports, we can all track patients, and we all have electronic medical records at this point. It's really, like I said, that continuity, that consistent relationship that changes health care. (Uma)

Accessibility involved both a physical and emotional presence, that is, having patients believe that even when not in the presence of their doctor, they could get a hold of them and receive a response back to their concern in a timely manner. This fed into the accountability aspect, which was not only key to developing trust in the relationship, but also helped doctors get to know their patients better and provide greater continuity of care over time.

I'll give some of them [my patients] my cell phone number, and I will get text messages or phone calls, even when I'm not on call. Which is risky, because you don't want to get burned out and constantly have people calling you, but so far so good. That accountability, it makes you delve a little deeper into the patients' problems, psychosocial problems, not just lab work and what you see on the surface. It gets just a little bit into what their life is like—what their home life is like, what their jobs are like. (Uma)

Continuity is valued by people. Certainly I think you get a richer sense of who the person is and can over time provide better care because you know the person in the context of their family and all that stuff. (Wilma)

Some physicians, but not all, believed that the electronic health record facilitated their own ability to be accountable to the patient and provide care continuity, even within a fragmented delivery system where patients might not get to see their personal physician on a regular basis. This was the most important positive use of information technology cited in the study, namely, its use as a knowledge transfer device to buttress the relational bond between physician and patient, by acting as a tool that updated personal physicians in real time about other care their patients had received.

> If they call me at 10:00 on a Friday night, I can pull up their record at home and even if they didn't see me, say, "Oh you saw Dr. Johnson and he gave you this and you're having oh, that side effect. OK, well maybe that's, you know, not the right drug for you or, you know, whatever." I can immediately plug into what's been happening with them and then put the note in the chart saying, you know I talked to so and so and she had problems with this drug and I'll put that in her allergy list or adverse list. I think patients absolutely appreciate that. (Betsey)

The use of clinical teams also was discussed favorably by some physicians as a vehicle through which, in the course of busy workdays, patients could get their doctor "channeled" to them via their social interactions with staff such as medical assistants and nurses. In truth, there was a split, almost paradoxical view among doctors on how the use of teams and other health care personnel could help fulfill the accountability goal in this regard. On the one hand, some doctors believed strongly that patients were largely interested in having access to them as opposed to their support staff. This feeling was not stratified by physician age or workload. Rather, it was randomly distributed across physician interviewees. Alternatively, other physicians felt that non-physicians with whom they worked could function as "extensions" of themselves—plug-ins who interacted with patients in their (the doctor's) name, allowing the physician to experience less direct contact with the patient but still feel the latter received relational care.

> The good thing is that they [patients] know that Amber [a medical assistant] works with me, and if they get a phone call from Amber, and she said that I spoke to her, or sent her a message, and asked her to do this or that, patients know who she is, they know who I am, so there's a fairly high level of trust in that interaction. And so, that, I think is pretty much as good as a call from me, other than the fact that she can't always handle the questions that they may give back. (Steve)

Established teams with stable people, those tend to engender trust with patients. You're getting a phone call from a familiar person, for example, and I think that's reassuring for folks. I think that's a good thing. (Olivia)

Alternatively, some doctors expressed a potent realism regarding how specific types of "innovative" clinical workflows, which used team care as a central component, and were designed to push as many visit transactions through the office on a given day, might undermine their relationships and trust with patients.

> You have to be careful. If I am running over or too many things are coming up in the visit, what I say to my patient in that room is really, "I want to do this justice. And I know I didn't book enough time for it. And my bad, I'm sorry I didn't realize, but to do this justice, I've got to have you come back." They [the patient] seem to do OK with that. But now if it's happened a couple times and I'm double-booked on the day they come back, or whatever, that's just a disaster. They don't believe you twice that you care about them. They'll believe it once. (Maggie)

> If we move to a model where I'm more or less poking my head in at the end of a visit and saying "Any questions"? "Are we all good"? I do think that will change the dynamic and those patients won't look at me as their doc as much anymore. Doesn't matter who else sees them during that visit. I'm not so sure they're going to think of me as their person. (Billy)

E-mail communication between the patient and medical office also presented a mixed bag from the perspective of how it impacted the doctor-patient relationship. For example, several physicians interviewed pointed out that given an increased inability to see their patients in person whenever the latter wanted, and given personal preferences not to have their offices open on evenings and weekends if possible, e-mail communication brought with it potential benefits for holding together relationships virtually, and for letting patients feel that their physician was only an e-mail message away from them, even if was just for emotional support.

> I have a patient with dementia and she has type 1 diabetes. She's 60, so she's had diabetes for 50 years. She's getting closer to the end of her life and she has been married to this guy for 40 years and he now has—he's assumed more and more caretaker duties as she is starting to lose her memory. I've known them for 10 years. He's so burnt out from taking care of her and she's now at a point where she really can't take care of herself, so he's doing a lot of it. He's so frustrated and mad at losing his partner to dementia and his own life to her needs. So he e-mails a lot, and a lot of it's just, "Hi, doc. I want you to know she fell again in the shower last night." Because what's he supposed to do with that? A lot of it's just his frustration. So it's a little bit of a rant. I can't see him every day. I can't see him and I can't see him at 11:00 p.m. or 1:00 a.m., which is often when he's writing. But he's able to send off a couple of e-mails and I'll write back to him the next day or whenever, depending on how urgent it sounds. But he's able at the time that there's a problem to get it off his chest or ask a question. (Mary)

WHAT PHYSICIAN VIEWS OF THE RELATIONSHIP MEAN

What can we make of this seemingly resounding commitment among physicians to viewing *relational care* as the bedrock of a strong, effective, and personally satisfying doctor-patient relationship? Encouraging? Naïve? Inaccurate? Pandering? As we will see in the next chapter, this is increasingly not the type of relationship most patients feel they have with their doctors on a consistent basis. In an important sense, however, it is consistent with the literature discussed in the latter part of Chapter 1, which touts the benefits of features such as trust, communication, listening, and other interpersonal dynamics for various beneficial patient outcomes. To a person, the physicians interviewed believed that trust was what made a doctor-patient relationship work. It was the bonding agent connecting them with their patients in ways that allowed for better care delivery. It was the ethical foundation of the doctor's ability to act in the patient's best interest. Trust was also a feature established through the presence of other relational elements typifying doctor-patient interactions such as accountability, friendship, listening, respect, and dialogue.

To return to an earlier point, these physicians construed meaningful relationships as emphasizing the human elements that in their eyes were best nurtured organically through ongoing social exchange and multifaceted role-playing with their patients. There were no shortcuts or gimmicks, at least in hearing physicians tell it, with respect to building and maintaining strong ties with patients. It required meaningful doses of time and contact with a patient to gain an experiential reservoir of moments where patient stories were heard and discussed; isolated bits of knowledge about patients could be connected together; serendipity in discovering things about each other as people could be afforded; and repeated instances of validation for the faith each party had in the other could occur.

For all of these doctors, it was not the advertising of a credential for themselves or their practice that fulfilled this relational ideal and produced interpersonal trust. It was not their personal *brand* or the feeling of a strong buyer-seller relationship that made the difference. It was not the competent meeting of explicit obligations, the cornerstone of a retail approach, through activities like the correct implementation of a disease checklist or electronic health record. It was not even the adept enactment of their technical or diagnostic skills. Rather, it was the ability of two people to come together and understand each other well enough so that one of those people could see that there were efforts being made to meet his or her real needs and the other could feel significant personal worth in contributing to that goal, even if she or he did not do it perfectly or fully.

Dyads, Relational Care, and the Current Delivery System

Physicians defined their best relationships as *dyadic*, or person to person, which is an important point to consider in the age of corporate medicine, which places faith in things that undermine dyadic care, for example, lumping single patients into homogeneous groups; using information technology to create "low-voltage," network forms of communication; and delivering care through teams rather than doctors as single professionals. It comes up against, at least in primary care (but increasingly in other specialties), the decreasing emphasis on doctors interacting directly with their individual patients for more than the small amount of time when the physician's knowledge advantage and experience is needed for "closing" diagnostic and treatment decisions.

Through a dyadic lens, doctors envisioned their best patient relationships as in some ways akin to how we might view relationships between individual family members or close friends, albeit with a lower degree of emotional intimacy involved (although depending on how close one is to friends and family members, the emotional intimacy between some doctors and their patients may be relatively significant). At the same time, physicians emphasized their role of expert advisor, which coupled with the desire to feel friendship ties with some patients gave them a complex but personally rewarding set of expectations to manage on a patient-by-patient basis. Accountability also loomed as key for doctors. As they described here, to doctors accountability in the one-to-one relational sense involves being personally available at the right moments for patients. It is validated through longer and more uncertain social interactions, some of which will pay immediate dividends for patients and others that will not, but all of which lay the groundwork for future discoveries that aid diagnosis and treatment.

Though personally appealing and possessing a fair amount of face validity given that features such as trust resonate with the average person, this emphasis on the interpersonal dyad is misaligned in key ways with the larger delivery system in which physicians now work. It is also out of step with retail thinking, which emphasizes instrumental rather than relational behavior and believes more in the system than in any one individual to meet consumer expectations and needs (see Chapter 3, Table 3.1). These are not criticisms but rather statements of fact. Much of what we are now doing in health care delivery *de-emphasizes* dyadic relationships, and it may be said that the same holds for other industries and aspects of our lives. For example, the rise of social media and sites such as Facebook promote greater emphasis on maintaining networks of "weak ties" between individuals who have low familiarity, levels of intimacy, and emotional connection to one another (Granovetter 1973). This reality undermines the notion of "strong tie" dyadic interaction, which produces deep interpersonal trust between people, greater loyalty and tolerance toward one another, and better understanding of individual situations.

A few thoughts here are warranted. First, the very relational elements physicians valued as most critical are difficult to measure and standardize, or to capture fully in terms of how they contribute directly to better care outcomes or dynamics such as greater patient engagement in their health. This is because they are often both distal in proximity to beneficial patient outcomes and intermingled with other causal factors. For example, the explicit value of trust between doctor and patient shows up intermittently, such as when patients who have been depressed or experiencing stress for some time, and hiding it from everyone around them, experience a moment with their doctor in the exam room when they feel like opening up.

This moment may occur well after the patient has begun experiencing depression, perhaps months or years later, and other factors such as appropriate access to the physician and perhaps implementation of a good screening tool have created the relational opportunity. Yet, it remains only an opportunity until the physician who is trusted by the patient asks questions, listens carefully, probes knowledgeably into the emotions and psychology of the patient, empathizes with the patient's life situation, and creates tailored recommendations specific to that individual's capacity to follow through on them. It remains an opportunity only until the patient feels able to tell the physician his or her story, which doesn't happen without a strong connection between the two. All of these dynamics are difficult to quantify in the moment, or to fully comprehend with certainty how they will lead to the patient getting help for depression and improving his or her quality of life over time. For each patient, the likely outcomes will be somewhat different, rather than reducible to an easily specified benchmark.

Those who look at relational care as more quixotic argue that in a system with access to evidence-based medicine, "big data," and powerful analytics (e.g., through electronic medical record technology and sophisticated population-based algorithms), why must "quality care" and "value" be so dependent on these less transparent intangibles that continue to rely heavily on idiosyncratic interactions between physicians and patients? They state that even if everyone agrees that these elements are vital for good clinical outcomes and doctor-patient relationships, how can they practically be assessed, compared, and incentivized across *millions* of relationships? As physicians understood, it is simpler to assess, compare, and incentivize their behavior on whether or not they perform various screening (e.g., colonoscopy) and lab tests (e.g., hemoglobin A1C), or if they can assist in getting the blood sugars of most of their diabetic patients under control. This is part of the "dumbing down" of doctors' work—the complex not easily measured gets overlooked, and the cut and dried gets all the attention.

Within the current health system, things such as relational trust between doctor and patient are of less interest to stakeholders such as insurance companies, Medicare, policy makers, and others complicit in the metric fever gripping U.S. health care. They also hold less interest for the consultants, think tanks, and managers earning their keeps off of redesigning systems for greater efficiency or transactional speed. But activities such as listening well and engaging in meaningful dialogue in the manner physicians think important cannot be reduced to a single workflow step that is perfectly specified and timed, carries no waste, and relies chiefly on information technology, any more than a difficult conversation with a partner or child can be stripped of its emotion and wedged into a 15-minute time slot. In fact, listening and dialoguing may be two of the more inefficient dynamics in the scope of human existence. If doctor and patient know each other less well, these features become even more time consuming.

Thus, in a health care delivery system working to enhance the predictability associated with "quality" and "value-based care," prioritizing less predictable aspects of medical care seems a hard sell. Consistent with retail thinking, it might instead be better to simplify "good care delivery" through attention to more precise, process-oriented markers such as waiting times, adherence to clinical guidelines, and unnecessary hospital admissions. Critics contend that care elements like trust are too complex, too messy, and too particular to specific situations and relationships to be of much value for making bigger decisions around things like reimbursement. Instead, the argument goes, make communication as ritualized and prespecified as possible, such as that embedded in a standardized electronic health record template that instructs all doctors on which questions to ask every patient, or groups of patients, during a visit. If doctors follow and fill in the template, they earn reimbursement and bonuses. If they do not, then they must report that to the payer and suffer the consequent penalty. Increasingly, moving off script is not in the physician's best financial interest, particularly in primary care.

The Lonely Struggle to Be a Relational Physician in a Corporatized Health System

A doctor-patient relationship best realized as dyadic, and relying on interpersonal trust, communication, empathy, and mutual respect for its efficacy has less need for the types of innovations sprouting up around it in the everyday health delivery system. Innovations in which much time and resources are being invested, and to which powerful corporate interests are beholden. This point suggests that a strong doctor-patient relationship is not in the best interests of organizations and entrepreneurs interested in making over health care delivery using cheaper approaches that rely on virtual interactions and non-physician personnel. For instance, when a health system invests millions in implementing an electronic medical record (EMR) system throughout its organization, it does not want to hear about how many doctors believe that EMR is either a hindrance or a nonfactor in their ability to provide the best, most personalized, and responsive care to their patients. Instead, they want physicians to use the technology extensively and in a manner that drives down the expense side of the balance sheet, while also allowing the organization to connect more directly with patients.

Other innovations face similar physician neglect through a relational lens, producing additional organizational angst toward doctor-patient relational dyads. Regarding the use of teams, some physicians interviewed did see other personnel with whom they worked (e.g., the "team" broadly defined) as helpful in holding together their own (the doctor's) connection with patients, especially at times when direct access was problematic. But notably, few physicians talked about other team members as anything other than temporary extensions of their own established connection with a patient. Most physicians did not view their support staff as workers who might on their own develop direct bonds with patients that allowed them to work somewhat free of the physician's gravitational pull on the patient. Instead, they construed the team as a necessary vehicle for helping alleviate the administrative requirements now present in care delivery; as a workflow facilitation device to get through the day in a timely manner; and as a repository for the scut work that surrounded each and every patient visit. Such a more limited, physician-centric view is not how the rest of the system increasingly sees the team model. The rest of the system sees health care teams as direct competition for the traditional doctor-patient dyad model.

The implications of this misalignment between the direction in which our health care system is headed and the perspectives on relationships physicians have outlined are profound. First, consider physicians. A number of surveys show many are increasingly job dissatisfied and burned out, as well as skeptical of trends such as metric fever leading to real improvements in their work (Ryan et al. 2015; The Physicians Foundation 2014). In a recent large national survey (The Physicians Foundation 2014), three-quarters of doctors were pessimistic about the future of the medical profession, and over 80 percent felt the medical profession was in decline. The majority would not recommend medicine to their children or other young people as a profession, and the majority would retire today if they could. Perhaps most telling beyond the attitudes expressed is that many physicians are reducing their access to patients through cutting their own hours and closing their practices to new clients. These results hold across all physician ages, employment types, and gender.

A little bit of hyperbole in these types of survey findings? Perhaps. But even controlling out for some exaggeration by physicians, it still staggers the mind that one would find so many unhappy, disillusioned workers in what many would say is still the most prestigious, autonomous, and well-compensated profession on earth. Could the increasing discrepancy between what doctors value as important in the performance of their roles and how the health care system is evolving be behind much of this collective angst? It is as logical a conclusion to draw as any, especially when these same surveys consistently show that doctors care a lot about their relationships with patients. If 20th-century American health care let physicians to do what they pleased, the 21st-century health system is intent on limiting their power and influence. One source of power and influence for doctors is the ability to cultivate and maintain bonds with their patients, to understand them as unique persons, and to interact with them in ways that produce deeper loyalties and transcend the organizations and systems in which both entities are now embedded. In this sense, good relational care between doctor and patient may weaken the health care organization's influence.

What is alluded to here is important to consider for the number of implications that spring from it. For example, it suggests that doctors may be dissatisfied and underperform with respect to team care or electronic medical records (EMR) when they believe it is lessening their relational connections with patients. They may not fully be aware they are doing this, but nonetheless it would be a natural human response. Alternatively, health care organizations may push these disruptions onto physicians in part to limit some of their influence with patients. Given evidence that physicians now spend an inordinate amount of visit and overall work time attending to the EMR, there is little doubt it undermines their capacity to act on relational features such as listening and dialogue (Shanafelt et al. 2016). This lack of available time for relational care, coupled with a compliance mentality of needing to "check boxes on a list" may convince them that emotional connections with patients are less important to establish, and demotivate them to "go the extra mile" in developing the kinds of patient relationships they know work, but which involve features that are time consuming and highly unpredictable. This possibility is discussed further in Chapter 6.

Most importantly, the emotional intelligence physicians need to engage in relational care may wither on the vine because it is neither rewarded in the marketplace nor seen as a particularly good thing for improving efficiency or quality. Doctors may get fewer chances to cultivate relational skills such as listening, asking questions, empathizing, or knowing when to enact the friendship role and when to push patients as the expert advisor. For younger, inexperienced doctors fewer opportunities to grow these skills may make them less effective as clinicians, and increasingly unable to bond with their patients. All of them may grow somewhat disenchanted and cynical, perhaps toward their own patients, particularly the ones who need relational care most, because they understand that standardized medicine does not necessarily serve these kinds of patients well and for doctors to do so, they must work against how the system seeks to reward them. These realizations and psychological states can filter into many negative outcomes.

But what of patients? What about their views on the doctor-patient relationship? Are they aligned with their physician partners in emphasizing the importance and ingredients of relational care? Do they experience such relationships firsthand, and do they come to see the features embedded in relational care, such as trust, as the most effective and personally satisfying? If doctor and patient views are aligned, perhaps it bodes well for a return to some relational basics and perhaps a sidelining of retail-based approaches. But if they are not, then it fuels questions about the importance of the doctor in tomorrow's health system, the future of relational care, and the type of delivery system we might get in place of this more utopian ideal. The next chapter explores the patient view with these questions in mind.

Chapter 5

The Tyranny of Lowered Expectations

How Patients See the Relationship

For patients, the best relationships with their doctors involved the very things doctors identified as important, namely, trust, listening, emotional bonding, friendship-like connections at key times, mutual respect, accountability, and a physician who served as an expert advisor. As with physicians, trust loomed as the key overarching feature implicit in much of what they talked about.

> If you don't have that trust, everything is lost. You might as well find a new doctor if the trust isn't there. I think that you have to be able to relate to your doctor, to see them as someone that's not just your doctor but also is someone that you can discuss important issues related to your health. Where they also feel a need to provide you objective information rather than withholding stuff because they don't feel that maybe they can say it. (Teddy)

There was a stark consistency as patients related anecdotes about the most fulfilling moments experienced in their own care. Equally emphasized, regardless of whether it was a healthier or sicker patient, younger or older, was the value placed on feeling that they were important to their doctor as *unique persons* with life circumstances relevant to understanding their particular health status, and for how their physician might add value for them. They wanted attentiveness in this regard, that is, a physician who related to them in ways that, even if the relationship was new, felt deliberate, personal, and caring.

> Man, we talked about everything—everything; stress, mental health, family history, my job, my coaching, I mean just everything else like snowboarding, running triathlons, what I'm eating. I mean the guy [my doctor] went down a list of stuff and he was engaging. You know what I mean? Like he engaged—it was a great conversation for me to have with him. I had a stressful fall semester at school, teaching and coaching. And he was encouraging me to sort of take some steps to become less stressed and to get on the path of recovery from those two months that were very, very stressful for me. That's what really stuck with me, there was this emphasis on wanting me to get balanced after a tumultuous two months at school, and I put a lot of pressure on myself. He was open to that understanding, and he was more concerned also with now that you're 50, here's some stuff you want to avoid and that you want to make sure that your stress level doesn't get out of control because he knows that my family has a history of heart disease and stroke and diabetes. Frankly, I don't have any of that, but he doesn't want to see me have that either, so that was a really good conversation. I came away thinking man, that guy, he was concerned about how stressed I was. It was more the mental part of my health than anything else. Now because he knows so much about me and my lifestyle, I think he's going to be able to connect the dots a lot easier. You know? I see him as the guy who's going to give me the diagnosis that I haven't figure out for myself. (Cliff)

> I really value not feeling rushed. I really like when the doctor is thorough and not necessarily waiting for me to ask questions, but is trying to prompt me and figure out what's going on with my health, because sometimes you don't know that something's not normal. I like that my doctor will ask me questions. For me, I didn't expect that my doctor when I told him I was having problems running would be like, "Oh, well, then we should do this asthma test. Maybe

you have allergies. Let's try this out. Use this inhaler for a week while you're running and see how that makes a difference." I think that it could have been much more easily shrugged off, but he made me think that maybe there was something more to it. I thought maybe I don't do that well in the heat or something like that. But I appreciated that he really wanted to get to the bottom of it because there were lots of things that I would never have thought about. (Bette)

She [my doctor] specifically brought me in to help me understand the numbers and identified a couple of things that confirmed some of the things that I was experiencing. She said, "We're going to work on this together." My mouth dropped. She said, "We're going to meet monthly, and we're going to work on this together." I had a little bit of weight loss, and she was celebrating that on the computer. She turned the laptop—the famous laptop—around, and she said, "Look when you were here a few weeks ago and look now. You're already in a good place. If you do this and you do this and you do this, I'm here with you to be a part of this." I could have cried. I think I almost did. Just because for my life space and the needs that I had, she was hitting all the right buttons. She was inviting me to come back monthly, which was a little wild to me. It definitely felt as though she had my interests in mind and that she had a goal in mind for me, and that she was going to do everything that she needed to do to help me get to the goal that I set for myself and what she saw in the numbers. Completely different experience. She would ask, "How are you feeling today?" Not like, "Are you sick?" It's like, "How are you feeling today? How's life going?" Things like that. It was just a very unusual conversation, but extremely aligned to what I was looking for. She was masterful at it. She asked those kind of questions like, "How are you? How are you feeling? How are your stress levels? What is causing stress?" It was almost a little like therapy at the beginning in some ways. She was definitely trying to get my behavior. "What do you do when you wake up? How are you getting the kids out the door? How do you commute? How do you balance exercise and commute? Because it sounds like you have no time." She did a lot of that, and that immediately bonds you to somebody. And then out of that, I was able to illustrate some of my complaints. She had a context for which those complaints were occurring within. Again, they weren't complaints that were dire, on my deathbed, but they were complaints that probably are pretty common of a 40-year-old mom with several kids and a big commute and a big job. But yet she could connect that and then be able to turn it around and take a look at certain areas of my care and be much more cognizant of where it might be stemming from. And she remembered. When I went back, she recalled some of our conversation and all I can think of is she had a system to note take. She wasn't doing it in front of us, but she remembered. It was like coming back to an old friend. It consisted of more qualitative questions to get me to open up and for her to get a sense of who I am. Versus the questions where they just throw at you and you're just answering against the back of a laptop. Very, very different behavior. (Janell)

My old doctor acted as if she knew me, and I believed it. I felt like I had been there often enough that she actually truly remembered these things. Whether they were or not—maybe they were well-placed on the screen or whatever. But I didn't feel like we were going down a checklist. I didn't feel like she was asking, "Okay, how is your this? How is your that?" I felt like she was asking open-ended questions and letting me talk. It was more of, "So how are you feeling in general?" As opposed to a specific disease or something that she's referring to. (Hallie)

I'm 27 and I actually just switched primary care physicians recently because I felt like I wasn't getting the attention to care that I wanted or needed. Before I was kind of rushed. Or just that my old doctor wasn't really paying attention to my needs. Just kind of like a one size fits all for whatever I went in for. I felt the attention that I was given definitely changed and my new primary care physician actually took the time to get to know me since I was a baby so that probably helped a little. She [my current doctor] got my background so she could diagnose better and to get more of a larger picture of what was going on. She was just really thorough when I saw her for the first time and all the things that I brought to her attention she tried to address the best that she could. She also followed through on things. She sent me follow-up paperwork. She sent me to a dietician. Because I kept on going to her saying that I'm tired. And at my old primary care they were just saying, "You're just getting older. That's just a part of getting older." Which I understand but I felt this doctor took the time to listen to me and investigate things rather than just slapping their assumption on it. (Tonya)

For patients, "quality" clinical care and a physician who sought to relate to them on a human level were the same, similar to how physicians saw it. Patients did not highlight, at least where primary care doctors were concerned, the importance of technical skill or a deep reservoir of medical knowledge as the deciding factors in whether or not they experienced a personally satisfying or effective relationship. Most already assumed that every primary care physician was properly trained up to a point, and as we will see, where they felt something was beyond their doctor's ability, they emphasized a role for the specialist physician rather than hold it against their primary care doctor. Instead, for primary care doctors what patients wanted sitting before them in the exam room was a trusted person with whom they could identify; one who sought to gain knowledge not through prefabricated, standardized questions asked the same way of everyone, but rather through a serendipitous face-to-face exchange in which the physician's approach at that precise moment ebbed and flowed with the patient's revelations about his or her everyday life. In this sense, they valued skill, but it was *interpersonal skill*, the kind not born from book smarts but rather out of an interest in learning about one's patients, seeing them for who they were, and feeling personally accountable for their well-being. Again, this was very much how physicians saw the situation.

Of course, patients talked about the best relationships with primary care doctors in terms that on one level might be seen as the result of not understanding the technical aspects of "good medicine." In other words, one explanation for their consistent highlighting of the softer relational features as important might be that they simply were not better able to discern the instances in which their doctors applied clinical acumen in incorrect ways, or used the differential diagnostic process inappropriately. But it was more than that. Although as non-clinicians we are limited in how well we can judge the purely technical side of medicine, the patients interviewed spoke with a robust confidence about their knowledge of the relational side of medicine. To some, it was articulated as common sense, defined and discussed without hesitation. For others, it was presented more as a set of elusive dynamics that they did not think about too much, but when asked to remember those physicians who had made them feel best, came out almost as fond memories.

Although the core features of an effective, personally satisfying relationship could be articulated by patients, many also stated quite clearly that they did not currently have such a relationship with any physician. This was surprising given the passion with which some of them spoke. In fact, only a handful of patients interviewed believed they currently had a high degree of ongoing relational care with their primary care physician. These were a mix of individuals with well-established doctors and ones who recently had begun seeing new doctors. Others spoke from past experience with particular physicians, or they referred to isolated moments with physicians they remembered, but moments which had not been strung together over time to create, in their minds, a fully satisfying relationship. This meant that at least some of the relational features, such as trust, that patients valued did not necessarily originate from a deep pool of personal experience. In this way, as with some of the physicians interviewed, it was unclear when patients' views reflected a more abstract, romanticized notion, based on personal dogma, about what doctors should be like, and when these views were firmly grounded in the crucible of frequent direct contact.

This lack of ongoing relational care also conveyed that the features patients said they wanted and valued, namely, trust, dialogue, respect, empathy, compassion, listening, and accountability were more situational for patients as compared with doctors. This made the desired features generally seem simpler and less theoretical in terms of how they could manifest in the everyday clinical setting. It made it seem as if there were fewer excuses on the part of doctors for not being able to exhibit them, given that the latter were not holding physicians to a standard that depended upon years of ongoing interaction. While physicians conveyed in their discussions that good relationships and trust took time to build, patients were more forgiving of the time investment required. For many of them, it was not about having every moment of their interaction with doctors come across as highly relational in nature. It seemed more about having singular moments of emotional bonding and personal attentiveness that felt real and not orchestrated. Anything more than that was great, but this was the minimum bar for them.

Through the interviews, it became clear that patients increasingly understood, at least from their perspective, what their doctors could and could not do for them on the relational side. For example, many patients knew about the ways in which their doctors used care guidelines and checklists in their interactions with them. But overall there was less sympathy for the physician's plight, or for the larger delivery system in which they worked. First, patients saw through the "checklist care" that frustrated them and that physicians increasingly seemed (in patients' minds) unwilling to stop in their daily practice. Second, many patients, particularly younger ones who had never known an ongoing relationship with a single primary care doctor, had come to believe that what these doctors and this part of the system could do for them was limited, and that included the ability to provide relational care.

Increasingly poorer experiences trying to access their physicians directly convinced many patients that perhaps the primary care physician was not as important to a good care experience as they might have presumed. In addition, the less than amiable workings of many doctors' offices, set up in the patient's mind to obstruct rather than to assist, nurtured the conclusion that relational care was at best sporadic and often serendipitous, for example, the product of a kind physician going the extra mile rather than something purposeful built into every fiber of medical office culture. These beliefs, fed by a bubbling spring of transactional care experiences flowing ever faster, shaped patient feelings about the prospects for personally satisfying relationships with any doctor. In short, patients did not come across as optimists where relational care was concerned. Instead, most of them were either pessimistic or ambivalent about their relationships with doctors, the result of several lowered expectations discussed next.

THE TYRANNY OF LOWERED EXPECTATIONS: WHAT PATIENTS TOO OFTEN GET WITH THEIR DOCTOR

What was idealized through various anecdotes as the best kinds of doctor-patient relationships got juxtaposed in patients' minds against the lowered expectations almost all of them had with respect to the total relationship quality they experienced with their primary care doctors. It should be noted that with few exceptions patients believed great relationships were not necessary with *specialist* physicians. Instead, for that brand of doctor, the expectation was almost pure technical competence, that is, addressing a narrowly focused clinical issue correctly, quickly, and with good skill application.

My expectations of a personal relationship are much less with the specialist. I'm there to get their specific expertise and get somebody who's knowledgeable about a problem that has been identified. I don't have an expectation that we will get all warm and fuzzy and that sort of thing. (Hadley)

I went in there [to the specialist] with the goal of trying to get pregnant rather than the goal of fixing a health problem for me necessarily or evaluating my general health. It was like I knew something was wrong, and I went there to fix it. I did have different expectations, and I expected them [the fertility doctors] to have less bedside manner and to be more technical, like "This is what we're gonna do. This is how we do it." And that's exactly what they were. (Bette)

I cut off the tip of my finger. I had to go to a surgeon, and it was just more of like, "Here's what's going to happen." It was very dry, and he spent a lot of time going over his surgery. But there's zero emotion, and even to the point where—it was funny, because the way he was trying to tell me about my emotional well-being and what the emotional reactions were going to be, it was so dry and deadpan. Like, "Here's what's gonna happen. I'm gonna put one stitch in it. You're gonna go home"; and he explained all the reasons for that: "It's gonna start to heal back. We don't wanna go in and do the skin graft until after that process starts. Your surgery will be at 6:00 in the morning," and it was very detailed. And then right in—towards the end of that, he's like, "Also, it's important for you to understand that in an accident like this, you're probably gonna have some depressive episodes. You're gonna feel like, 'I'm such an idiot,' and that's perfectly normal." I couldn't tell if he was trying to be caring. But that's not primary care, like you'd hope that someone that you're working with on a repeated basis, like a primary care physician, would have more of an understanding of how you might react as an individual. (Edward)

This left primary care physicians as the doctors with whom the majority of patients saw the features of relational care, like trust and empathy, as most appropriate. That said, the lowered expectations they expressed sounded depressingly familiar. It also was consistent with the notion of a health care system in which primary care doctors and patients are hamstrung to interact the way they prefer and see fit. For instance, almost all patients were ambivalent about proactively cultivating emotional bonds with their doctors. None came across as feeling able to be proactive. Nor did they feel that doctors could pursue their own agenda in this regard. Rather, there was a grudging acceptance that the more singular moments of relational excellence still experienced from time to time were exceptional rather than normal. I began to feel myself during interviews that these high relational moments were so vivid in some patients' minds precisely because they stood out against the backdrop of the normal everyday delivery system—shallow, evaporating watering holes within the arid interactional deserts shaped by transactional care delivery.

I think the biggest change is now it's become more mechanical, more computer, less human interaction, less discussion. It's a rubric-based system. Before my doctor would sit me down and talk to me actually eyeball to eyeball where you felt that he cared and he checked my history, he checked my results, he talked. Since that doctor retired I have gone through two or three primary care physicians personally because I felt as though they don't care. My physical exam used to take 45 minutes. My physical exam now takes less than 10. The difference being the interaction time, the lack of getting to know me, like what are you doing, what type of exercise do you do? That's what I used to get. The probing questions and the history of me. I feel the medical field now has gone away and lost that personal contact, whereas before you had that personal contact. They embraced your sickness. They embraced your well-being. They embraced you for who you are and stood by it. (Rich)

You tend to go into all this now with low expectations, because the experience has led you to believe that's all you're going to get. Everything from the aesthetics of the office to the experience you have when you're in there leads you to believe that you are one of many, and that you have 10 minutes on the calendar, and that's what it is. Just "tell me what's wrong and here's the prescription". (Janell)

It's being treated like a human being. Even feeling like I had a quote, unquote "decent relationship" with my PCP, you still felt like you're going through like a processing plant. I mean, it's like you go up. You take a number. You fill out paperwork. Somebody hands you a clipboard, "Go sit over there." You do that. There is this feeling that you're just being shuttled through. (Edward)

The place I go to now is a little better. The last doctor I went to, you were a task, not a patient. (Grady)

A few older patients who had been with the same primary care physician for years, and who believed their relationships were adequate, were still apprehensive about the future. They talked about seeing warning signs with their doctors related to things such as the physician's time availability and increased adherence to standardized care. They also saw real changes occurring within the medical offices they visited, and talked about them in ways that reflected a genuine puzzlement as to why things were moving in certain directions. Younger patients were less apprehensive and more accepting of the status quo. They had a smaller set of experiential reference points to draw upon in believing they had been exposed to high levels of relational care in their past. For them, that type of care was simply more randomly obtained, so its loss or absence seemed less personally offensive to them.

The lowered expectations most patients had of the doctor-patient relationship took the form of several different beliefs. These were that primary care physicians: (a) were increasingly firewalled from them and less accessible in a timely manner; (b) were interacting with them in truncated ways that were too "generic" and driven by a feeling of "checklist care"; (c) could do fewer things for them because of perceived competency limitations and their lack of knowledge about them as unique persons; and (d) maintained operations in their offices that were ambivalent to treating them as valued customers. Such beliefs formed a common understanding among patients of "patient care today" and, as we will see at the end of the chapter, they enhance the potential for disruptive innovations that bring with them retail thinking and a view of patients as consumers.

Patient Aversion to Checklist Care: Seeing Through the Facade

Despite the current notion that standardized care delivery, in the form of checklists and clinical guidelines is good for us, patients did not see it that way, especially when it came to primary care medicine. One of the strongest findings in the study could best be summed up as a strong patient aversion to what often was described as "checklist care." Checklist care involved anything physicians did in the course of care delivery (e.g., a face-to-face visit, virtual communications between doctor and patient) that appeared (to the patient) too generic or standardized, or was perceived to go against the desired treatment as unique persons that patients claimed they wanted. What was striking, for example, was how many patients referred to the same behaviors across different physicians in this regard, including doctors "reading off scripts"; "asking the same questions over and over"; and "not looking up from the computer screen."

My biggest pet peeve is to just get off the script, and listen to what I'm telling you, and we can save ourselves both a lot of time. I had actually, through some early career stress there, lost a decent amount of weight. I think when I graduated college, I was like 195. I was like 185 within nine months of working. He [my doctor] was like, "Oh, you're in the above-average range. You might want to lose a couple pounds anyway," and it's just that disconnect, so I say, "I'm really stressed out. One of the manifestations of that is I'm losing weight, and yet you're telling me that I'm overweight." It didn't feel like a good fit in terms of the kind of attention to my personal need. It was much more of, "Well, let's go through all the general questions." "Let's go through all the standard things that we would do in a normal initial kind of meeting with a primary care physician—blood pressure, cholesterol, full labs, all that stuff." But I just did not get a good vibe that this would be somebody that I trusted to work with. (Edward)

There's a little bit of a recognition of me as a person but nowhere near what the sort of interaction there was in the past. It just seems a lot more business-like now, like I'm there just to help her fill out her forms about me. I value it because it's a regular follow-up and it's a full-fledged doctor, but I don't have the close personal connection I want. (Darlene)

Even for complex patients suffering from one or more chronic diseases, where standardized care through the use of checklists and guidelines is more accepted and beneficial in guaranteeing a minimum level of quality care for a specific patient population, there was concern expressed with too much interaction along these lines. At least from these patients' perspectives, standardized care delivery through the application of a disease management guideline was not necessarily meant to better serve *them*. These patients talked about how they wanted physicians to spend a good deal of the time, especially in the increasingly rarer moments of face-to-face interaction, dialoguing about how they were personally managing and coping with the effects of their diseases, and how their particular circumstances either helped or hindered their ability to have an appropriate quality of life on an everyday basis.

They also wanted their doctors to probe more deeply with an eye toward trying to find out what else might be coming down the road for them in terms of additional health complications or diseases. Many already were well-versed in "their numbers"—the hemoglobin A1Cs, body mass indexes, and lipid profiles. They understood both the significance of different levels for these tests and what those levels meant. These patients complained that, in essence, visits to their primary care doctors were set up more for the doctor's benefit, containing rote reviews of metrics, physicians and staff obsessed with getting them recorded, and nonstop rehashing of standard chronic disease management information known and no longer helpful (in the patients' eyes) to furthering their situation.

> I'd like to see my doctor not have to go over the same stuff every visit. They generalize and throw you into a group. If they knew me a little better, they wouldn't have asked me for a half-hour about a medicine for smoking cessation I've already been on. (Tommy)

For these types of patients, who are an increasingly large number in the health system, it was particularly disappointing given that at least upon first diagnosis of their disease(s), they were able to see their primary care doctors more frequently than other patients for face-to-face visits. This is because in the current delivery system, a sicker patient with a newly controllable disease gets immediate attention, due to a reimbursement environment that penalizes or rewards doctors for hitting the right metrics with respect to *groups of patients* who have a given disease. Yet for these patients, more visits did not translate into greater relational care. Instead, they talked about how each visit often felt like the one before it. The feeling of a *generic* approach to their ongoing care left some of them lamenting missed opportunities, such as the doctor learning things about them specifically that could be important to improving their health. Hallie and Will were patients with several interrelated chronic diseases who captured this dynamic. Hallie had been with her doctor only for a few years. Will had been seeing his doctor for a couple of decades. This difference in the length of relationship didn't matter.

The doctor that I have is even more transactional and very seldom looks up from her computer when she's talking to me, and it's more filling out a questionnaire that she has pre-programmed in there. I answer the questions, and obviously if there's a flag she picks up on it and refers me out if she needs to. I would say that she doesn't ask any follow-up questions, for one. If she asks a question and I answer it, if it doesn't trigger something in her brain that maybe could need further study, she's moved onto the next one, and she doesn't have me elaborate at all. She doesn't look at me, for one. She's staring at the screen during the whole thing, and her fingers are moving. Unless I say something that is outrageous—I think I could say there's a purple elephant in the room and maybe she'd look up. But other than that, I don't think she would. I actually think, in some ways, she also failed me a bit, because I had diabetes for probably a year before she picked up on it. She was looking at probably my weight, my general health, but still sort of missed that I could potentially have diabetes. And so I do think that conversations help—we don't know what to say that will trigger the concern, so sometimes you have to sit there and listen for a little while to figure out, tease out what the issues are. (Hallie)

I find him [my doctor] asking questions now more that he just . . . he's asked over and over again. I don't remember him doing that much. Each time now in he goes through the same things— I take four different pills, two for diabetes, a couple for other—a statin, blah, blah, blah. So every time I go there, rather than saying any change, he goes over each item individually, even though it is current. I don't know quite why, maybe he has to check it off on the computer. I don't remember ever doing all that, he used to just say "any changes?" that kind of thing. I just find him spending much too much time looking at his screen and asking me these questions. (Will)

The push back here might be that because the chronic disease patients interviewed were somewhat knowledgeable about their diseases, and part of a cohort characterized as better educated, such disappointment around care delivery that in their minds was too "cookbook" is less important given that many complex chronic disease patients may require a steady drumbeat of tests, "numbers," and standard guidance to help them navigate their conditions, either because they are noncompliant in their own care or simply less able to take a deep interest in their own health. Although perhaps accurate to some degree, the notion that patients need metrics thrown at them relentlessly to let them know if they are doing badly is a paternalistic view of patients generally, smacking of "lowest common denominator" care and understating the physician's imperative to know when, as Edward notes above, to "move off the script" and treat uniquely.

It also misses a larger point observed in how chronic disease interviewees captured their interactions with physicians. Chronic disease patients in the study were not dissatisfied that their doctors made sure "the numbers" were in order at each visit. They expected some of that and felt it appropriate to a point. What annoyed and frustrated them was that rather than make up only a small piece of the interactional moment, it tended to define it. They felt their doctors were beholden to the metrics rather than to them as patients. This perceived reality about checklist care lowered their expectations that face-to-face visits with physicians were worthwhile, which is ironic given that chronic disease patients were the ones needing to believe that regular visits with or input from their physician had value, given their diagnoses and potential for other complications.

The perceived overexposure to checklist care fed into other thoughts undermining patient feelings that strong relationships with doctors mattered. It made all patients wonder at times about the competency of the physician before them; conclude that the physician understood them better as a generic *one* of a similar group of people with the same diseases; and feel skeptical of the larger delivery system's desire to meet their personal needs. None of these thoughts were good, either for getting patients to believe that it was worth the effort on their part to bond with their doctors, or to feel that physicians cared about them in more than simply a quantitative sense.

I think doctors now have become so "get the people through" because there's many problems that they have to deal with every day that they don't think about you specifically. I've not met one that

thinks about me tomorrow. They're not going to think, "Oh, I wonder what happened with her" or something like that. (Winona)

Not Easy to See

The lack of accessibility to their doctors also lowered patient expectations
for the type of service experience they might expect, and whether relational care was a realistic goal. For younger patients with less prior allegiance to any physician, the lack of timely accessibility to see their primary
care doctor reinforced a belief that it probably was less important to have
a regular physician.

> Times when I needed a sick visit with him [my doctor], it was pretty
> hard to get one. I pretty much only use him for my annual visits, and
> then when I needed to have a sick visit, which maybe would happen
> once a year, they—his office staff—would actually just tell me that
> I should go to the urgent care center. (Bette)

> If I am sick it's usually not at a convenient time for a primary care
> physician's office hours, something that would work for me, so I go
> to urgent care. I don't really feel having a primary care physician is
> that valuable. I also feel like they don't have the time to treat the
> whole person, they're there to treat an ear infection, they're there
> to treat one specific problem and I don't feel that gets to everything.
> (Darlene)

> It got to be so hard to get in to see my doctor that I could get into
> urgent care quicker. So I got to know my urgent care doctor better
> than my regular primary care doctor. (Grady)

Almost all patients interviewed commented on being unable to see
their primary care physician face-to-face when desired. The most common
anecdote in this regard was the "I called my doctor's office and they set me
up with someone else to see" story, which when viewed from the health
system's (and physician's) perspective may be a normal part of redirecting
hectic workflows in the age of heavy demand, but holds a more profound,
if subtle, meaning for patients, that being—*you cannot see your doctor when*

you want, we [the medical office] can and will make that decision for you, and you have little ability to control it.

> I've had my doctor for three years. Only been three years. I saw him two years ago for my first checkup with him, and we went through everything, and he says, "Well, I'll see you in a couple years. You don't need an annual checkup. Every few years is fine." So my interaction with him has been pretty much, "All right. You seem to be okay. Let's check with you in a couple years, or as needed, but otherwise, let's not do too much." (Barry)

> You have to be strategic if you want to get in to see your doctor. My office, you have to call them at like 8:01 when they open, because they have same day release appointments. And you have to call right on the dot or you don't get it at all. If I can't get in that day, I ask them [the receptionist] when the next same day release appointments for my doctor will be, and she tells me the date, and I put it in my phone so I can remember to call. If I'm really sick, I then have to get my doctor's nurse on the phone to try and convince her to get a same day release appointment for the next day with my doctor, and if she agrees then she [the nurse] can release one for me. (Carly)

There were other aspects to the accessibility issue. Some patients worried about the physician "being there" mentally for them even when the two parties were face-to-face, as well as the increasingly short interpersonal interactions between doctor and patient that defined primary care. Patients spoke of distracted doctors in the exam room; too much interfacing with medical assistants and nurses instead of the physician (i.e., the "health care team"); and consistently shorter physician face time than anticipated.

> You're in a room alone for 90 percent of your visit. Seven of the other 10 percent, you're with a nurse or a clinician, and then it's like you get a couple minutes like with the doctor—"What's going on? Tell me about it. How's this? This is what I'm doing. Let me verify that he or she did what they were supposed to do," and then you get moved on. (Edward)

I spend a lot of time with people who aren't the physician. The medical assistants, nurses, everyone but my doctor. (Mia)

They also spoke of a lot of inconvenience in terms of the long waits and paperwork completion that preceded their interpersonal contact with the doctor. Generally, every patient interviewed presented portraits of their "normal" interactions with primary care physicians that contained some degree of significant disappointment. This constant exposure to subpar service delivery in one or more forms upped the level of criticism toward doctors.

I don't want a few minutes, and I don't want to have to wait an hour and a half to get that few minutes. I wanna know, like can I come in there at 9:00, that you're mine from 9:00 to 9:30, whatever it ends up being, and we're gonna talk about me, and you're gonna be prepared, more prepared than what you read in the minute of looking at the chart. (Rich)

If my doctor saw me in the waiting room, she wouldn't know who I was. (Tommy)

Most patients expressed feelings ranging from ambivalence to outright anger toward the manner in which some physician offices were set up to operate on a daily basis, in their minds a setup often intended to make their experience trying to access the doctor even worse.

This whole idea that you're not a customer—it makes me crazy. When I go into an office, and it really doesn't matter whether it's my pediatrician or the women's health doctor or the internist, these frontline people are lacking. They act like they're stressed out, and they act like they're overworked, and I'm sure they are, but then that comes off as you don't have time for me. It's not a great experience. (Siobhan)

I hate going to the doctor. I hate sitting in the waiting room and feeling like I'm going to catch something from somebody else, and that I'm waiting there forever. I feel like more often times than not, office staff can be pretty incompetent or rude. (Susan)

There's a certain type of receptionist that you find across the board. Very seldom do you find someone that is actually very helpful at the primary care level. I have not found that. They seem to me like they're overworked, don't like their job. Very seldom do you have somebody that has a caring sort of demeanor about them. There's always places that have disgruntled employees, but you can tell if someone's overworked or pissed off or expected to do more than they're supposed to do. It comes out of them, and that's how they handle you, and they have that already in their head. I would say the way I've been handled has been surprisingly similar and consistent across different doctor offices. Like a waitress, you can tell when they're serving you food either they're happy to see you or they're not. And that's the way you feel in a lot of these primary care offices, there are people that just seem like they're not happy with their jobs. (Hallie)

Lack of timely accessibility and a growing estrangement from the doctor convinced several patients that interacting with the larger health care system was perhaps more trouble than it was worth, resulting in patients who preferred to either ride out basic illnesses without trying to gain access to a physician's office, or avoid preventive interventions such as annual physicals.

I used to have pretty decent physicals. Then they went to this other type of physical where the blood work was like, "Oh, you don't need this; you don't this, no big deal." And I'm like, "Well, what is my physical then? What if my white blood cells spiked for some weird reason and I felt perfectly healthy, but now I have some underlying cancer that's growing. Now I'm not gonna know for another year." Because I feel good. Fifteen minutes for a physical. When four or five years ago, it was like a good hour. And we had a good conversation. Now I don't feel like there's a benefit to get the physical. I haven't even made my appointment for my next physical. I just was like, "Well, maybe I'll just wait two years." You know? Even though I'm at the 50 marker. (Raul)

From Relational to Transactional: Patients' View of the Primary Care Doctor as "Traffic Cop"

Whether it was the lack of direct accessibility over time, producing patients less knowledgeable about what their primary care doctor could do, or some other factor at work, most patients in the study concluded that primary care physicians could do less for them than they preferred. This lowered expectation made some of them wonder about the value of needing to access them in the first place, much less trying to cultivate a deeper, ongoing relationship. Both healthier and sicker patients felt that bypassing primary care and going directly to specialist physicians was almost always an appropriate decision.

> If anything gets too complicated or too involved I'm seeing the [specialist] docs. And then I definitely get a sense that I'm dealing with people that are very knowledgeable in their particular areas. (Hadley)

> I recently had an issue with my asthma and I had to go to an urgent care [center] and then usually if I go to someone for like asthma and allergy issues I feel like I still have to follow up with my asthma doctor because I feel like the primary care doctor isn't as versed in asthma as the allergy nurse and doctor is going to be. I always follow up with my specialist just to make sure. (Tonya)

> My expectation is you go to a primary care practitioner for a checkup, but you don't go necessarily if you're experiencing specific symptoms where you know that there's someone else out there who can give you more information. I think that some people form these sort of implicit schemas in their mind of their local practitioner, that their general practitioner is going to be able to direct them or help them in every single way, shape, or form which they need. I think that we're living in an age in which there's so many specialties and so much information, that that's just not possible. (Teddy)

> I think I've adjusted my expectations to the fact that they [the primary care doctor] really won't be able to help me with the chronic issues that I have, nor will they be able to identify problems. Once

you get into chronic problems, you tend to find the real doctor out there that knows how to handle it. (Hallie)

I feel like primary care has been becoming more limited because people want to go see specialists, and that means primary care offices aren't dealing with the kinds of things that they used to. I think just from knowing that, if I broke a bone, or if I needed stitches, which should be within the scope of primary care, I don't think I would go to a primary care doctor. I think I'd probably go to the ER, because I don't think that doctors in primary care see as much of that anymore. (Susan)

This crisis of confidence in the primary care doctor's technical ability, as noted earlier, did not affect patients' ideal of what the best relationships consisted of with these doctors, because that ideal was built on softer interpersonal features. But it did create in patients' minds a desire to access specialist physicians at any and all times for clinical problems that they understood as more involved, including select chronic disease situations. It was here that some patients emphasized the primary care doctor's role as "traffic cop" as the most important manifestation of the doctor's current value. Being a traffic cop meant serving as a resource that could help a patient (a) get to the right specialist doctor quicker and with less hassle; and (b) navigate other complexities of the delivery system, including getting necessary ancillary services such as testing, imaging, or physical therapy.

Being a "traffic cop" sounded like an important role for serving patients. When describing it, however, none of the relational emphasis came out in patient discussions. Rather, the traffic cop role was expressed in highly transactional terms, that is, as a set of straightforward exchanges between doctor and patient, some of which further undermined the legitimacy of the primary care physician as someone who was a "one-stop shop" for patients and their symptoms, as well as a trusted advisor and confidante for helping to assess clinical situations. Instead of a one-stop shop, the traffic cop role denoted primary care doctors as a *first, quick stop* on the way to other doctors and parts of the system, easing patients' ability to get *somewhere else*.

I appreciate my current physician can cut through red tape and get me all the right paperwork and get me lined up with whatever follow-ups [to specialists] need to occur. She's on top of all that sort of thing. I guess the bureaucratic part of it, which can get hairy. It's important that there's sort of an efficiency to the process so I don't get bogged down. (Hadley)

I think my feelings about primary care changed the minute I had to ask them to go see other doctors, years ago. As soon as I saw that doctor [the primary care doctor] in order to see another doctor [a specialist physician], it set up the expectation that I have to do this [visit the PCP] to get somewhere where I need to go. Instead of thinking of the primary care doctor as where I'm going for my health care, I'm thinking, I need to take this step—this annoying step—to get to where I really do need to go. And I think mentally, once that happened and I saw that this was just something I had to do—I stopped seeing them as their own entity, and that they could actually solve my problem. I saw them as a stepping stone. (Hallie)

I assume that they [the primary care physician] are the first starting point for your care. They are physicians that are kind of the directors of traffic. I don't expect them to know anything deeply, because I assume that anything surface is very routine. (Janell)

Of course, being a traffic cop for help in navigating the rest of the delivery system is typically cited as a key aspect of a primary care doctor's job. It comes with various labels, such as "care manager," "care coordinator," and "medical home." But it is portrayed as only a smaller part of the primary care physician's overall value to the patient. What was more disturbing about how these patients talked about the doctor as traffic cop was that such a role was not discussed in the context of other more sophisticated roles such as doctors might play for patients. It was not an additional role these doctors played alongside other more relational ones, nor was it a role that involved any sort of deep involvement by the PCP. Patients did not articulate it in the spirit of believing that their primary care doctor could deliver on a range of more complex care delivery or the relational care promise, or that their doctor was easily accessible. Instead, for these patients it was presented as perhaps the only viable function their primary care doctor could play for them now, that is, getting them "where they really needed to go."

This narrowing down of the primary care physician's role also opened the door in many patients' minds to using non-physician providers such as nurse practitioners (NP) for more basic primary care service delivery. The lack of timely accessibility to primary care doctors also fed into this reality. For example, patients perceived NP's as easier to access, in part because their experiences in the system convinced them that it was true. They also felt such non-physician providers perhaps could deliver basic primary care medicine as well as physicians.

> I would be hard pressed to differentiate between the nurse practitioner and the doctor as far as knowledge and experience and involvement and all that stuff. (Hadley)

> I think it comes from my experiences with both, which have really been the same experience across the board. Whether it's a physician, a nurse practitioner, or a physicians' assistant. They've all been able to do the same things, or I've gotten out of the visit what I needed to every time. I don't really see a difference besides the initials they have after their names. (Darlene)

> Can a doctor do a Pap smear or a breast exam better than a nurse practitioner? I don't think so, I really don't. I think I'm more astute than the majority of the public in these sorts of things; maybe it's because I did grow up with a doctor as a father. But I definitely never approach a relationship with a doctor as, "They know all the answers," because they don't. Certainly my nurse practitioner has never steered me wrong. And I have had a great, long-term relationship [with the NP]. (Siobhan)

> The nurse practitioner does everything that the primary physician does. Again, because it's all transactional. It's rashes. It's ear infections. It's the same kind of thing. (Janell)

This increased exposure to non-physician providers gave patients more transactional rather than relational care experiences because non-physician providers tended not to have specific patients assigned to them in such places as urgent care centers, retail clinics, or even doctors' offices (their normal places of employment). There simply was not the expectation that relational care through ongoing visits with the same provider would be provided in many of these settings. Many patients spoke with a grudging reluctance about having to orient their own mindset toward singular visits with NP's and PA's in which convenience was achieved, but fewer relational features, such as trust or accountability could be, given the compartmentalized, often very brief, nature of the interpersonal exchange.

THE NON-RELEVANCE OF TECHNOLOGICAL INNOVATION FOR RELATIONAL CARE

Finally, patients discussed the role of technology in helping or hindering relational care with their doctors. Perhaps the most important finding in this regard was that no patient believed the most common technologies now being used in doctors' offices, including electronic health records and electronic patient portals, contributed meaningfully to better relational care with their doctors. Patients did not come across as against the use of such technologies per se. Rather, they had few experiences of real value that they could convey in terms of where such technologies enhanced relationships with their doctors.

Doctors relayed the usefulness of virtual communications at select times, for example, in helping to maintain relational features such as accountability, communication, and trust. Patients, however, did not highlight this same usefulness, which was somewhat surprising given the rhetoric within the health care community related to the benefits of information technology for "patient-centric" care and consumer engagement, and the significant financial investments being made in health information technology within doctors' offices. Generally, patients seemed ambivalent about the role of these technologies in their care delivery, while expressing in particular some worry about too much use of them within the exam room itself.

I think the only thing for me, and perhaps it's one of my worries, is how far this experience is going to go with the interviewing and the laptop situation in the examination room. To be honest with you, I have experienced it to the point where it's intrusive in the 10 minutes they give you. (Janell)

It seems like most of his [my doctor's] time with me is spent just trying to get everything into the computer, while they are still trying to talk to me. Like there's so much stuff they need to get into that thing. He tries to look me in the eye and not make me feel like it's intruding, but then he still keeps pecking away almost the entire visit. (Mia)

Interestingly, the more ambivalent view that electronic technologies do not add much value to the doctor-patient relationship was not specific to a single cohort of patients, such as older patients whose prior experiences with doctors for years had been without the presence of these innovations. Ironically, some of the greatest ambivalence came from young patients who had been immersed in smartphones, personal computers, and all things electronic since their childhoods. Tonya was a patient in her twenties who typified the younger view.

Physicians are moving towards using the laptop instead of pen and paper and I feel like that totally disengages them from the patient. I know we're moving one way technologically and it's probably easier than having somebody enter it all later but I feel like that's taking away from the interpersonal relationship between the patient and the physician. My doctor will apologize. He'll say, "I'm sorry. I'm not ignoring you. I have to type it in [to the electronic record]." But it just takes away from the flow of the conversation. It makes for a different dynamic in the room. I know him and I know that he cares about me as a patient but it's still like every time I'm talking about my symptoms and stuff usually he's typing or clicking drop down boxes. That takes away from the experience. (Tonya)

Virtual communications, in the form of electronic "patient portals" that most primary care offices now use to varying degrees, and which theoretically could connect with patients once outside of the office, were seen by a number of patients as more trouble than they were worth. Several different reasons accounted for this belief. First, they were perceived as logistically difficult to navigate in most instances.

> My doctor uses a patient portal. I don't think anyone likes the patient portal. I really don't use it just because I find it an annoyance and yet another pain in the ass. A set of passwords to remember. I don't use it at all. I usually use him [the doctor] for a sounding board more to kind of maintain my health and I don't see a patient portal really as being helpful to me in doing that. (Matt)

Second, a number of patients talked about how the kinds of information normally placed in an electronic portal or record were difficult to understand.

> The portals are the only thing that I've probably experienced, and then the electronic results [e.g., labs, tests] through those portals. I have no idea what my passwords are. I have no idea how to find my results online. Literally, I'm lost every single time I go onto it. I find them to be frustrating because they're not intuitive. They send you your [test, lab] results and it's in Greek. You have no idea what you're reading. So it's sort of useless. Send me the results, but if it's all in Greek, I'm not going to have any ability to interpret it. (Janell)

Third, some patients, even younger ones, accustomed to interacting in a variety of highly transparent electronic realms with few privacy protections, did not trust these technologies to protect their information.

> I feel like there's a lot of great things that technology can do but I just don't know about my health information being online and being able to access it. It's great that my labs are online, that's cool I guess, I don't know. But you see all the time about patient information being hacked and stolen. I also feel like sometimes too much information is not good information. Everyone can't decipher labs. (Tonya).

Fourth, some patients felt that doctors themselves were not bought into trying to use these technologies to enhance their relationships or connections with patients:

> I've been told [by my doctor], "Oh, I never check that." I was actually told by my primary care doctor that I shouldn't leave notes there [in the electronic portal], because they are not checked regularly. So I kind of gave up. She said that if I have anything that needs to be responded to within 24 hours or whatever, just to call. (Hallie)

> If I were to login and go into the portal, then I could find information. But it's not like they're [the practice] shooting out mass e-mails or something like that, saying like, "Hey, you haven't logged into the portal in a month. Come and check it out," that type of thing. (Rebecca)

This is not to say that the use of technologies designed to allow doctor and patient virtual access to each other and to important information will not grow more popular in the future. A number of patients did state that in theory they liked the idea of being able to communicate with their doctors electronically. But the question of *expanded use*, which seems to be more the preoccupation of policy makers and health care organizations currently, is not the same as the question of what such technologies might do to *enhance relational care*, that is, features such as trust, dialogue, empathy, accountability, and mutual respect. Even the doctors who thought the technologies had some value for maintaining particular relational features cited small, less impressive examples of them actually delivering this value. For both patients and doctors, then, it seemed as if electronic health records and patient portals, serving as the advance guard of additional innovations coming in the future, simply were not that relevant to building and sustaining a personally satisfying relationship between patient and doctor. In short, none of them saw technology in any form as something that at present really mattered much in their assessments of the best doctor-patient relational moments.

WHAT PATIENT VIEWS OF
THE RELATIONSHIP MEAN

In hearing the patient's voice, certain things come through loud and clear. Some of these are consistent with how doctors think about their relationships with patients. Others reflect a pragmatic stance suggesting less possibility for strong relational bonds with doctors. This pragmatism is fueled by lowered expectations about what is possible for doctor-patient relationships and why. These lowered expectations loom as key threats to maintaining patient mindsets that see doctors as able to provide meaningful relational care on a regular basis. They imply a version of the future for doctor-patient relationships that could involve one group standing pat (doctors) and another making reluctant but profound changes that lessen the dyadic importance of doctor-patient interactions within the overall health system.

Overall, patient views of the doctor-patient relationship suggest that they could be the group to provoke these changes in the future. For example, they may be open to new forms of health system innovation typified by the retail philosophy and its emphasis on transactional quality. This focus could satisfy needs for timely access, convenience, cheap care, and system responsiveness, at least on paper. On the other hand, there is enough reading between the lines in the evidence presented to also assert that patients may not be as willing or ready to embrace innovations that reflect more of these transactional imperatives. For instance, patients did not come across as overly "engaged" in seeking out new innovations for their care, or assuming control over their health. Quite the opposite, they talked in reactive tones about what they saw as uncontrollable events occurring around them; events many did not care for in their health care lives. In short, with few exceptions they did not appear to be anywhere near the kinds of proactive or engaged consumers we might see in other walks of life. They were increasingly ambivalent about the value of primary care doctors in their lives, and seemed to be moving through a mindset change that weakened their own long-term desire to fulfill the ideal of strong relationships with doctors.

Similarities and Differences Between Patient and Doctor Views

Patients and doctors see eye-to-eye when considering the characteristics that define personally satisfying, mutually beneficial relationships with each other. The consistency of viewpoints between the two groups is compelling. When asked to define the "best" experiences with their doctors, patients identified those same *human elements* of good social interaction that physicians also made clear were most important. These elements included trust, listening, emotional bonding, friendship-like connections, compassion, empathy, mutual respect, physician accountability, and the physician as expert advisor. Most of all, they valued relational moments in which doctors treated them as unique individuals with specific histories and circumstances. Their best moments with doctors were ones, as described, in which the latter showed interest and skill in getting to know them on a personal level, even if only briefly, taking time within the moment of a face-to-face visit to dialogue and acquire specific knowledge that could be used to provide tailored guidance.

It should be noted that none of these elements were specifically prompted by the researcher. I did not ask patients to tell me how important trust or accountability was to them in their interactions with doctors. Rather, similar to physicians these qualities emanated from the mouths of patients as they described their best experiences over time. To hear about their importance to patients in the context of smaller anecdotes lent them an authenticity that was typical also of the physician perspective. Like doctors, patients focused less on the technical acumen of the primary care doctors with whom they interacted and instead on the interpersonal skills these doctors brought to the table. In their minds, a strong, effective relationship centered on face-to-face interactions of a high quality, interpersonal nature with their physicians. It was *dyadic* in nature, as doctors also emphasized.

That patients and doctors shared similar perspectives on the importance of these relational features is not surprising. After all, most of us crave and benefit from things like trust, respect, and being treated as individuals across the entire spectrum of our lives, from school to family to jobs and friends. We benefit from making emotional connections with one another. In one sense, why would health care be different? We seek out health care services and interactions with a physician at some of the most vulnerable moments in our lives, and when we know something may be wrong with our physical or mental health. Many of us traditionally have gone to primary care doctors for in-depth appraisals of our health status, and to pull from us submerged feelings and information about our lives important to predicting our health. Whether we know it or not, all of us yearn to tell our story to someone when we feel sick or hurt. But to deliver on these intents, the features both groups identify as important must be present in abundance. Thus, the two stakeholders directly involved in giving and receiving care, even without a lot of experiential evidence, know intuitively that relational care has value.

That said, the relational features identified by both groups are not things insurance companies, government agencies, policy makers, or industry executives seem to prioritize all that much right now. For example, much trust in the industry remains calculatively (through pay for performance) rather than relationally cultivated, leading to less focus on the quality of the social interactions between doctor and *individual* patient and greater focus on paying doctors to follow specific clinical guidelines and meet standard quality targets for *groups* of patients. If anything, the current system increasingly incentivizes stakeholders to keep individual patients *away* from physicians, especially with respect to face-to-face care. Such interpersonal care is expensive and in the eyes of many often unnecessary, driving up short-term service use in the process, even as other intangible rewards are provided for both groups through such care, and long-term costs decrease as health conditions are discovered or anticipated through regularly occurring, intimate probes of patients' lives and circumstances.

There were also key differences with physicians in how patients captured their best moments with doctors. For example, the patients in this study sounded as if they had at their disposal a smaller number of prior experiences seeing the relational features noted above in action. Although it was also likely that some physicians had smaller sets of strong relational experiences, the nature of their work seeing dozens of patients each day likely gave them more interaction moments where the benefits of relational care could be potentially evidenced. In addition, their experiences presented as more longitudinal with specific patients, and they certainly emphasized, at least in theory, how important getting to know and interact directly with a given patient *over time* was to solidifying strong emotional bonds.

Alternatively, patients thought such relational features could be experienced in "real time," whether or not doctor and patient had a longer-standing relationship already, or had interacted in a highly relational way previously. As we saw earlier in the chapter, the majority of their anecdotes relayed the features as occurring in a situational, sporadic manner. Whereas doctors emphasized the extended time and repeated contact it took, for example, to cultivate features such as trust and accountability, the patient perspective was that many of the features required a lower bar of interpersonal intimacy for their manifestation. To some degree, both groups romanticized how important these features were for themselves and good patient care. Patients, however, were less dogmatic in when and how these features could manifest with their doctors. They just seemed grateful for the times when they were present.

Lowered Expectations and the Potential for Retail Approaches to Take Hold

The views of patients and analysis presented here suggests the presence of already damaged doctor-patient relationships. Somehow, I got the impression when speaking with patients that good relational care was the serendipitous, single drink of cold water they got occasionally on a hot day rather than the permanent, predictable, and free-flowing unlimited supply of hydration they accessed at their discretion. After all, patients also conveyed clearly that the best interactions with their doctors, as defined by the presence of the relational features discussed, was increasingly not realized for them when seeking care. Only a handful of those interviewed, approximately 15 percent, conveyed any type of stable, long-term relationship with their primary care doctor.

But even long-term relationships with the same doctor did not guarantee that deeper connections with patients had been established. The remainder of patients spoke of their primary care doctors in a variety of different ways that often conveyed both a physical and emotional distance from them, despite occasional moments of relational care. For instance, some patients spoke of never seeing their "regular doctor" except for physical exams once a year. Others spoke of newer relationships with their doctors in which neither party seemed to know much about the other, and noting that there simply wasn't enough time or direct contact to improve the situation. In addition, patients saw specialist physicians as pure technicians providing a high level of clinical expertise and surgical skill, and not expected to deliver on significant doses of empathy, dialogue, respect, or friendship. Relational care from specialists sounded more like a luxury add-on than a necessity. Alternatively, the physicians interviewed made it seem as if deeply relational bonds between all doctors and patients—primary care and specialists—was a good thing, and beneficial. Again, theirs was a more universal take on what a "doctor" could establish with any given "patient."

Although attention to the viewpoints of both doctors and patients around how to transform care delivery is arguably limited at present, there is no doubt the patient view is absent in greater magnitude when it comes to policy debates and managerial interventions around the types of "care innovation" the health system should be pursuing. Summaries of generic surveys like CAHPS show that almost half of primary care patients believe that their doctor does not pay attention to their mental and emotional health during a typical visit, yet they also show that many patients seem satisfied with their doctor visits. What do these paradoxical results mean? Satisfaction with a visit in the absence of good relational care is not all that surprising, as patients can think they are "satisfied" for any number of more superficial reasons. These surveys usually ask about individual *visits*, not ongoing doctor-patient *relationships*. Visits are highly transactional generally, and many patients may think about their satisfaction with aspects of the transactions that occur (e.g., did the receptionist handle your information correctly?), rather than their holistic relationship with the doctor. Thus, some may feel satisfied because they got the prescription or specialist referral they wanted, some because the receptionist was extra nice to them. Others might be satisfied because the physician did not run late that day and saw them on time. Still others might have gotten better by the time of survey completion, attributing improvement in their cold or their sprained ankle in part to that particular office visit.

The patient view expressed here, namely, that good relational care may be conceived of as more sporadic and "in the moment," suggests that the bar has indeed been lowered for many patients in terms of what they expect to see when receiving care. Maybe a patient who thinks a doctor has actually listened to them for one minute of a visit, or asked them questions about themselves for another minute is providing good relational care, and should be trusted. But relational trust inevitably grows strongest from longer-term interactions; a build-up of common experiences between two individuals; and validation that one's personal vulnerability is not taken advantage of by the other party over time. It cannot be fully realized within single visits of short duration with strange physicians or health care teams in which other relational features are evident for only brief instances.

What is perhaps most concerning about the patient perspective presented here is the potential confusion some patients may have between *real* relational care and singular moments of doctor-patient interaction that have relational features, but are not fully representative of deeper connections with a single physician over time. This observation does not bode well for the future of the doctor-patient *relationship*. It could support the growth of a vastly cheapened form of "relational care" within the health care system that rests more on style than substance—and allows system stakeholders, maybe even doctors themselves, to use relational elements in artificial ways that serve as ground cover for models of service delivery non-dyadic in nature, which are geared to maximizing transaction volume rather than interactional quality and meant to give everyone the same level of standardized care experience that is lower cost and more profitable for suppliers.

Although the findings presented here suggest a complicated road ahead for health care organizations interested in promoting consumer engagement at least in part through retail approaches, they also suggest that there are legitimate opportunities to create new ways of interacting with patients within the system. These new forms of interaction will rely upon a fuller appreciation for the range of individual needs and preferences beyond those built primarily on the bedrock of doctor-patient interactions or relational care. Understanding the implications of the lowered expectations described, as well as the continuing hostile care delivery context undermining physician-patient *dyadic* interaction, inform this assertion.

One viable scenario extends from the interview data. For instance, it could be that patients' lowered expectations toward getting relational care from their doctors leave them psychologically susceptible to having other expectations and wants imagined for them by health care organizations like insurance companies, hospitals, and retail-oriented companies like CVSHealth and Apple. As dyadic care with physicians is experienced less, patients (particularly younger ones) lose some of their collective memory regarding the value of relational care. This susceptibility plays into the hands of those interested in pursuing retail approaches that involve promoting *buyer-seller* relationships with patients; building and leveraging corporate brand to strengthen customer loyalty; and innovating to deliver new products and services, some outside of the health care sphere, and many not involving physicians, which get targeted to specific patient segments.

As patient trust in physicians perhaps grows scarcer, that trust becomes up for grabs, even as a more transactional or calculative attribute. Organizations with lots of resources, multiple established channels for distributing services and products, established inroads with patients from either past health care or other product buying experiences, and strong reputations could potentially garner some of that available trust. Imagine an increasingly dissatisfied or underwhelmed population of patients, frustrated toward physicians and the delivery system generally, and tired of feeling like mistreated widgets when receiving services. To the extent more of them feel less in control, and begin to pay more out-of-pocket through high-deductible insurance plans and larger copays, which is now happening, they could embrace more of those market-based values and expectations that typify retail thinking. They will become interested in trying out new services, perhaps in ways they had not previously imagined. Among other things, this could include getting services from non-physician providers and delivery outlets not controlled by physicians; using technological tools conjured up by organizations that give them greater personal choice in when and how to access care; and getting health care services as part of a larger buying experience that also includes the opportunity to purchase non-health care items.

An increasingly disgruntled patient can be marketed to with the promise of *something different*—grand pronouncements of improved service; unparalleled quality; lower out-of-pocket costs; and smaller things that somehow seem to fit what they as individuals think they need. The creation and targeting of these messages, derived from the reams of personal information health care organizations will collect from patients both now and into the future, is a particular strength of the retail approach, and so there is a very real fit here between seller strengths and buyer proclivities that could find deep traction in promoting a tighter purchasing bond between health care organizations and patients. Immersed in such a culture, patients as consumers also may begin seeing *health care* in ways similar to how they see other industries in which they interact, shop, and buy things—as a diversified marketplace where multiple sellers compete for their business on the basis of several equally valued features including price, quality, convenience, timeliness, and reliability.

But it will not be easy, if considering only the patient view, to enact such a reality in full. The lowered expectations described here, in combination with patients still believing that their best moments with physicians are dyadic and contain strong relational qualities, could work against the spread of retail thinking, at least in the short-term. For example, as features that are heavily interpersonal in nature, such as trust, listening, and compassion, start to grow less interpersonal, less physician-centric, and more broadly defined by the health care system, they will get co-opted by a variety of interests, in the process taking on different meanings that may not appeal to patients. Further value confusion and frustration on the part of patients could occur.

If the organizations promoting retail approaches cannot actually improve significant parts of the patient experience they are supposed to improve (e.g., convenience, access, timeliness, cost, quality), the darker underbelly of buyer-seller relationships could get exposed. This darker underbelly reflects the profit-driven orientation of retail approaches taken to extremes, exhibited through a coldly instrumental drive to turn patients into uninformed, superficial "buyers," of, for example, services, products, and ways of thinking about their health. It must also be said that the lowered expectations toward primary care doctors, as seen here, do not automatically imply that patients will dispense with a loftier, deeply personal sense of what they want in their health care experience. They may continue to crave highly interpersonal, relational care moments with doctors for reasons they may not fully appreciate, at the same time they also ask the system to meet these other expectations and needs. They may want to have their cake and eat it, too.

These two chapters have given a glimpse of doctor and patient views of the relationship at its best and most satisfying. They also have described the harsher realities pressing on these views; realities that both groups increasingly seem to feel are outside of their ability to change. But before we pass judgment on that assertion, it is useful to explore in greater depth the continued ceding of care to the health care corporation, through the eyes of doctors and patients—a process that threatens to remove physicians further from our view; make doctors and patients more dependent on organizational resources and goodwill for their survival; and lay further groundwork for the retail philosophy to take hold. The growth of corporatized care relationships looms as the biggest threat to relational care within our health system.

Chapter 6

Ceding Care to the Corporation

Making Doctors Disappear

The forces presented in Chapter 2 as transforming the doctor-patient relationship, namely, the health care quality machine taking over health care; value-based reimbursement for physicians; the proliferation of larger, resource-intensive organizational structures that oversee doctors; and the increased demand for health care services making transactional speed paramount are evident in the concerns doctors and patients express. As described in that chapter, they involve an ever greater ceding of care planning, management, and delivery to the large-scale corporation—whether it is one that directly employs physicians or one with whom physicians affiliate to better manage the administrative complexity they now face. All physicians, whether "self-employed" or "salaried worker" now adhere to a specific set of uniform requirements and standards in providing their services to patients, particularly in the area of primary care. Their workdays are regimented and increasingly prescribed according to the needs of their employers. The push to standardize care delivery in all its forms accelerates over time.

The modern health care corporation assumes primacy in this particular context for seemingly rational reasons: (a) the need to provide the appropriate resources and scale that pursuing the Triple Aim of lowered costs, improved population health, and enhanced patient experience requires; (b) gaining enough patients to spread the financial risk associated with value-based payments across a diversified population; (c) implementing reliable quality-improvement workflows that monitor, measure, and intervene; and (d) developing multiple care access points to get patients timely services. As both doctors and patients have implied, however, giving over important responsibilities like these to health care organizations impacts the doctor-patient relationship in meaningful ways, which, among other things, undermines the strength of the relational dyad between the two groups.

Two particular impacts are discussed in greater depth in this chapter. They have been touched upon in the preceding chapters through the voices of doctors and patients. But their potential effects on important levers of change such as the expectations patients hold regarding their care; who they may give their allegiances to in the care domain; and the ability of individual doctors to embrace relational features in their work, as well as execute on a more dyadic care philosophy, merit further analysis. The first impact involves how the various aspects of metric fever, quality monitoring, and care standardization—all gaining their legitimacy under the rubric of "population health management" (PHM)—undermine physician motivation and ability to deliver relational care. Through the various facets of practicing PHM at the primary care practice level, physicians not only become less likely to engage naturally and over time with their individual patients in ways that build emotional bonds and trust, but also are likely to grow frustrated with their situations, leading to further demoralization for some, and for others offering a pragmatic impulse to passively accept things as they stand. Both of these outcomes make doctors less useful as agents of proactive change in reasserting the tenets of relational care, and may make them complicit in placing the organization in a more powerful and controlling light.

The second impact involves the insidious manner in which the lowered expectations patients hold of primary care service delivery, specifically the recasting of the primary care doctor as a "traffic cop" getting them to where they "need to be," begin to shift patient loyalties away from the individual physician and toward the larger health care organization of which that physician is a part, and which now holds more of the "one-stop shopping" potential in terms of access to different doctors and other needed health services. Patients want relational care in their interactions with doctors, and know the positives such care may bring. Yet, this particular impact of shifting loyalties raises the question of whether patients are open to a redefinition of the construct of "relationship" in ways that involve the physician much less, the organization much more, and a reimagining of personal preferences and expectations that align better with transactional care delivery and the retail philosophy. This point was touched upon in the prior chapter, but it bears greater scrutiny here in the context of patients being immersed in a new normal of larger systems of care.

POPULATION HEALTH MANAGEMENT: THE ENEMY OF RELATIONAL CARE?

From the health system's perspective, and the organizations within it, a key facet of running things effectively in the age of corporatized medicine includes a heavy emphasis on "population health management" (PHM). PHM, a form of implementation for the larger ideal of population health talked about for years by public health advocates, is making its way into every aspect of U.S. patient care in the twenty-first century, affecting physician work (IBM 2016). Consider the following quote from the IBM Care Management application software web page, which describes a population-based health product:

> IBM® Care Management *is a packaged software application that delivers key capabilities required to manage care across the care continuum. It can identify clients in need of care, assess their needs, establish the appropriate care plan to support their needs, manage the care and monitor results and outcomes. IBM Care Management combines data integration, analytics and coordination of care capabilities into a single ready-to-use offering that offers a personalized, 360-degree view of the individual to facilitate outcome-focused care (https://www-01.ibm.com/software/city-operations/smartercare/solutions/).*

It sounds an awful lot like what we have always expected the physician to do for us, right? PHM involves the practical, everyday application of actions, tools, and strategies—for example, the use of standardized care protocols and guidelines, health information technology (e.g., electronic health records) to record and communicate, analytics that crunch data on lots of patients to form individual treatment plans, aggressive patient-segment care management—to seek lower costs, greater predictability in care delivery, and a minimum level of quality care throughout the delivery system. In its fullest form, though, the PHM philosophy also presumes to do a more robust job of managing patient care than individual doctors.

The beauty of PHM lay in its potential to create a more transparent, equitable health delivery apparatus. The danger of PHM taken too far involves, among other things, seeing patients less as individuals and more as faceless members of larger clubs, that is, clubs of specific chronic diseases, care delivery pathways, and health compliance behaviors. It is a concept that has yet to meet with sustained critique, and yet in at least one way it should. This involves the manner in which its tools and strategies threaten physicians' legitimacy with their patients, in part lessening the former's centrality in delivering relational care on a dyadic basis. In some respects, the effective implementation of population health management requires a heavier emphasis on good transactional care delivery—getting patients to do stuff, tracking groups of them, analyzing bits of "big data" to identify who needs tests and screenings, connecting patients with additional services for their particular disease profile—than it does on relational care. For example, one health care start-up recently came out with a computer algorithm, using medical claims data, it says can predict which types of patients will die within a year, for the purpose of identifying and better managing needed services for those patients (Beck 2016).

For doctors, PHM means learning to think about patients in terms of "things to do" with them, perhaps engaging in less quantifiable and financially rewarded dynamics such as "talking," "listening," or "empathizing." In the world of PHM, there may be little incentive to be good at relational care, because proving one is good at process-oriented care and "checking the boxes" may just be enough to get paid and acknowledged as an effective physician. It arguably does not depend for its success on how emotionally connected an individual doctor is with individual patients, how much face time they spend together, or how well that doctor actually knows a given patient. After all, those things serve in part to identify things potentially or actually wrong in patients and the right treatment approaches to consider.

If PHM tools and tactics claim to be able to do the same things through an algorithm or some other form of artificial intelligence, in theory, the individual doctor's tool box grows less necessary.

The rhetoric put out there by some is that a physician also is motivated to be good at relational care through a PHM lens. PHM and relational care are not mutually exclusive, they say. *Of course it matters.* But in the reality of time-crunched workdays; patients who churn through the delivery system with lowered expectations; team-based care and EHRs getting between doctor and patient; doctors and patients who spend much less face time together and know one another less well; and payment linked to excelling on standardized quality measures, why would this assertion be true? In such an everyday world, what are the workplace factors working *in favor* of relational care? Is providing "good care" to your diabetic patients by having their appropriate exams done, medications managed, and blood sugars checked dependent on relational care? Doctors would say yes, but PHM proponents would assert that more important than dyadic interactions between doctor and patient is the presence of a reliable data system within the medical office that can identify patients who are noncompliant, do not come in for visits, or whose A1C is above 7. Important, too, they would assert, is holding doctors financially accountable for reaching out to those subgroups of patients, and then giving those doctors canned tools (e.g., diabetes group education, on-site care managers who can aggressively track the patients down) to shift the averages within the subgroups of desired processes and outcomes to where the guidelines say they should be.

Many physicians interviewed seemed to acknowledge that the full realization of PHM in everyday clinical practice depended more on the resources and efforts of the larger health care organization than it did on their own ability to provide relational care to patients. For instance, they spoke with grudging acceptance of the need to have the organization at their side in order to meet, document, and report out the numerous performance measures on which their work was judged. They articulated how without access to the larger pool of resources and infrastructure needed for performing the various aspects of PHM required by payers and accrediting agencies, they would have less success in meeting the external goals around efficiency and quality placed on them.

Most physicians were aware of how the infiltration of population health management into their everyday work and interactions might disrupt their relationships with individual patients. For example, some talked openly about having to lessen their face time with patients so that other non-physician staff on the team could engage in the work of gathering quality-related information from patients and recording it into the medical record for later reporting. They described the application of rote questionnaires in directing their conversations with patients. Almost all physicians felt that their workdays had become overloaded with tasks that in their minds involved record-keeping and keeping insurance plans and accreditors happy. For some, the work of PHM seemed to lessen their motivation to pursue interpersonal relationships with their patients. In our discussions, though, it wasn't clear that they fully grasped the potential magnitude of this outcome, nor how the ever widening scope of PHM activities in their practice might further reduce their own influence with patients.

Physicians presented several points of contention in this regard. First, many of them implied in their discussions that a constant emphasis on meeting important but basic and numerous standardized quality metrics for their patients, a key tenet of population-based health management, could lead to changes in the interactional dynamic such as greater interpersonal conflict and frustration between the two stakeholders that lowered the prospects for trusting relationships. In speaking about this topic, one of the things that bothered doctors was their own knowledge that context and the individual's personal situation mattered. Yet, in their minds understanding such idiosyncratic information about patients was not considered a big part of the quality equation in terms of what insurance companies and Medicare paid them to do. Bobby, a family physician, provided the example of the annual Medicare "well visit" to illuminate this tension between the basic, standardized care requirements he needed to administer and more personalized patient care.

The Medicare wellness visit is something that's supposed to be better for Medicare patients, but it's really the opposite of what we've trained to do as doctors. There's no physical exam; it's basically a standard assessment of a patient's medical status. And on the surface, that sounds pretty good. We're supposed to review the medications. We're supposed to review the different types of doctors who they're seeing; we're supposed to try to totally coordinate that. We're supposed to review advance directives. We're supposed to do some simple screening for depression and for mobility and for functional status, but we're not supposed to dig for or address problems. And this drives patients absolutely crazy, because they're not there to have all this stuff assessed; they're there because they have problems they want heard and taken care of. I have a really hard time saying to them, "Well, I'm sorry, this visit that you've been scheduled for is for me to do all this other stuff; it's not to find or address your problems. We'll have to schedule you a visit to do that stuff." We belong to an Accountable Care Organization, and as part of our Medicare ACO we have got to have a certain compliance with these annual wellness visits. I have to do a certain percentage of them, or my organization stands to lose a lot of money. So we're getting a lot of pressure to do these. (Bobby)

Some physicians lamented a care environment where doing what was needed to "check a box" and fulfill the demands of an employing organization more interested in managing the care of patient groups placed them in adversarial postures with certain patients.

It's sadly misplaced faith in [quality] data that they [insurers] think that a person's hemoglobin A1C is an assessment of how good their care is. I mean we all know that we don't have control over that. And to pretend that we do, it just means that you're giving doctors incentive to give up on patients and say go somewhere else. Take my smokers. I've got smokers that would kind of come to this truce that they say they're not going to quit and I say okay, I won't bug you about it but we both know that I know that it's not the right thing for you. And we just stop talking about it, because if we keep talking about it, it destroys the relationship and so we kind of say OK, this is a truce on this but we'll work on this. (Betsey)

Like their patients, physicians were disdainful for the most part of the metric fever they now felt dictated too much of their interactions with patients. They seemed to know and appreciate what patients in the last chapter did—that too much "adherence to quality scripts" undermined relational elements such as trust and respect in the doctor-patient interaction. Added to this feeling was a concern about how using PHM tools such as electronic health records often took precedence in time-limited interactions between doctor and patient.

I don't know how much you've actually seen some of these things, but they're totally ridiculous. Like we have to do templates on all our chronic care patients and note whether we've spoken to them about what they need to do, and whether we've reviewed their medication with them and whether we've talked about the side effects with them and what kind of goals we've set for them; whether they should eat vegetables or not; whether they should smoke or not; or whether they have barriers to care. And on the surface, well, yeah, that sort of makes sense. Those are all things that one should be addressing. But from my perspective, these are templates that are imposed upon me that come up [in the electronic health record] at the end of my visit. I've either dealt with it or I haven't dealt with it by then, but I still have to answer the questions as the electronic template asks them of me. From what I understand—and I've actually sort of looked into this—I don't think that there's any evidence at all that these templates have done anything at all to improve the quality of care, but they certainly take time. I really resent that a great deal. Our institution can get them to pop up automatically, and there are more and more things that pop up all the time. So, for example, now I have to do a functional assessment on all my patients, including my children. And the assessment is: Can they walk? Can they not walk? Well, 95 percent of my people walk into the office. So they have no problems, yet I have to complete the paperwork for this. I make the argument all the time that we're a patient-centered medical home, but our front office, our telephone triage, stuff that matters, is miserable. So, we are not patient centric at all; yet, at the same time, we meet all the criteria that the government places for us, because of good paperwork and so we get that sort of designation. I think that that's a real problem. (Bobby)

Trying at times to sound diplomatic, physicians suggested in many conversations that gaining information on various aspects of care delivery for insurance companies and accreditors placed them directly in the middle between the insuring organization and patient; a place they did not wish to be. Besides placing them into potential conflict with their patients—pleasing the organization on the one hand versus pleasing the patient on the other—they simply felt it took too much emphasis away from giving patients other valuable attention they might need; attention less easily measurable and highly idiosyncratic to the particular patient.

> I feel like we would have a bigger impact for people and be able to provide them better quality care if we actually helped them with more social support and life advice than we did with making sure they had their Pneumovax. Sometimes we default more into just making sure that they had their flu shot and their immunizations, and forget the whole full picture. (Barbara)

> I have two jobs when I'm seeing a patient. One job is to take care of the patient, and the second job is to take care of the EMR, because I'm measured based upon how well I take care of the EMR. And I find that the two conflict pretty strongly. (Bobby)

Being put "in the middle" between payer and patient was a source of inner tension for some physicians, and of growing ambivalence for others about their specific role with patients. Both of these dynamics came out in how some doctors spoke of "noncompliant" patients in their practice, that is, those individuals who for various reasons were either not willing or able to be brought in line with what specific quality measures appropriate to their conditions required. These patients ranged from diabetics who would not take insulin or alter their diet to bring their hemoglobin A1C levels down to individuals past 50 years of age who would not get a colonoscopy to screen for cancer. Some of these patients had legitimate reasons in the eyes of doctors for not complying, while others simply exercised their personal autonomy in dictating their own health care trajectory.

Neither was acceptable through the lens of PHM, which relied on full compliance from everyone regardless of excuse—in part because of standard quality definitions but also because full compliance meant more accurate clinical and claims-based data sets that were used for further population health prediction and management. Although physicians stated that good relational care always called for a negotiated compromise between what they and patients wanted, having PHM thrust upon them daily made some doctors feel unfairly treated in that the less they could convince a patient to do something called for by a quality measure or clinical guideline, the more it was they who would be penalized.

> I do worry about the [quality] measures and how they reflect what I do. I've got patients who just don't believe in mammograms. They don't want to have a mammogram. And frankly, from what I'm reading, maybe that's not such a bad idea, but I'm still graded on what percentage of my patients have mammograms. . . If I have a big practice of crunchy granola-type patients who don't want to have mammograms, then that reflects poorly upon me. So, I've got to sort of report to the folks who collect the quality statistics, on the one hand, and then I've got to sort of take care of my patients and what they prefer or want, on the other hand. (Sam)

This caused some doctors to talk uncomfortably about their role as the organization's (e.g., insurer, employer) watchdog, that is, the point person for helping it get as many patients as possible to receive the same minimum standard of care as everyone else in their particular subgroup. This was an issue not easily raised with doctors. Some did not acknowledge easily the watchdog role. Other physicians had an awareness of its validity, yet struggled with how they saw it in their own minds, for example, as something which was overall either good or bad, necessary or unnecessary. Their defensiveness and unease came out at times.

> Sometimes I am a little more aggressive about making sure that things get done, OK? But I have not fired anybody from my [patient]

panel because they wouldn't get a colonoscopy, or I haven't gone to that extreme to say, "Oh, this guy's noncompliant, I don't want to see him anymore." I do have an increased awareness of somebody who hasn't had something done that I thought had something done. I think I'm a little bit more upfront with them, OK, about "Jeez, you know we really ought to get this," OK, you know? Again something more like a blood test, because the insurance companies are looking to making sure we're doing the right things for you and I think it's a reasonable thing to check. (Curt)

It's better if we're nagging people to get their stuff done. Nagging the people that don't come to attention that we can maybe get some headway on. Is it any better? I think we've got a whole new administrative burden to try to take care of stuff for people and it costs us a lot of effort and time. I don't know if that's better in the long run. I think we're all exhausted and spending less time taking care of patients. It looks good on paper. I'm not sure it translates into a lot of better stuff. (Burt)

TRANSFERRING WORK AND ROLES TO OTHERS

Feeling like a middleman or watchdog was one thing; abdicating direct contact with the patient and giving certain parts of patient-care work, even the most mundane of that work to others was another. The demands of population health management on their time and mental capacity to care for their patients in a highly interpersonal way was clearly apparent in speaking with doctors. Almost all said they were overloaded in everyday practice, facing a growing list of things to do around quality, care coordination, and documentation. As a result, many were increasingly letting their staff members, who were non-physicians and less trained, do things that traditionally they [the physicians] might have done directly or been more involved in as a regular course of action.

When my medical assistant comes into the exam room, she's making sure that you had your mammogram, your colonoscopy, and sort of filling those little check boxes that say we're doing good quality work. But when I come in, I still get to do the softer side, as opposed to reviewing all of the actual quote/unquote, "quality" pieces. (Barbara)

The medical assistants here own health maintenance. When they bring the patient into the exam room, they will go straight down the checklist and whatever they can do they will do. Mammograms, colonoscopies—the MA will actually book the patient for those things. So that when we [the doctor] come in to see the patient, we can maximize our time on the acute issues and not waste time on this other stuff. (Claire)

This work often was done by medical assistants and included taking vital signs, completing electronic medical record templates on patients, going through the list of required tests or screenings for a given patient, reconciling medications patients were taking, and initial triage regarding patient symptoms or reason for coming to the office. It also included interacting with patients virtually, through phone or e-mail, on requests to speak to the physician, specialty or lab referrals, and general care-management issues. Physicians spoke of this work and role transfer in straightforward ways, never raising the larger issue of how such transfer might undermine their own ability or motivation to maintain closer ties directly with their patients. They simply saw it as a normal aspect of the realities faced in their busy workday; one that was fairly benign in nature.

If I didn't have my MA do some of this more routine stuff, I'd have even less time with the patient. (Claire)

My medical assistant knows my patients as well as I do, and half the time she's so good that she will just call them and she'll be able to help them with whatever they need. I don't really need to be involved. She kind of lets me know later what happened. (Scott)

The patients come to know the medical assistants really well and it's just another part of their team. I had a medical assistant awhile back and she ended up leaving and a good number of my patients were like,

"Oh, where is she? We miss her." So they recognize her. They remember her. I think they see her as an extension of me, because sometimes I try to call patients back as much as I can but I'm only one person so I can't call everyone back. Sometimes, if it's something that I don't feel is life-threatening or really urgent, I'll give the message to the medical assistant to call back. The medical assistant's relationship with them helps me recall, like if I forget [something about the patient] I'll say, "When you go in there can you ask where they work." And they also have a different perspective sometimes than I have. The medical assistant has other experiences, other life stuff going on. Sometimes she can pick up on things that I don't or maybe she can add insight that I might not otherwise have. I also don't call my patients back personally anymore. I rely on the medical assistants to do that. (Rachel)

Besides work transfer occurring around the actual office visit, and also with patients attempting to reach their doctor by phone or e-mail with questions, physicians spoke about the active outreach and ongoing interactions with patients that other staff members, either working for them or, more commonly, for their employing organizations or patient insurers, now conducted. One manifestation of this is in the increasing use of "care managers" in primary care, particularly for those chronic-disease patients who have been branded difficult to manage. These personnel have become a key best practice in the implementation of good population health management, and it involves others besides the physician performing complex work with patients.

Well, our organization has the care managers for the complex patients, who will call and, at times, even go out to see some people with complicated medical needs, especially people in the Medicare group. The care managers can help to manage their care in the sense that they look and make sure that appropriate things are being done for them and see whether services might be worthwhile and just kind of reinforcing their compliance and behavior. (Curt)

So here's a different relationship. Those case managers I talked about, those people are RNs. And those RNs are people who I would send a patient to, say, "I've got a diabetic who's under terrible control."

I might send that patient to them with the goal of, "Hey, can you help get this person under better control?" And they might have all kinds of ideas from saying, "Hey, what do you think about starting some insulin with needles?" when I haven't done that yet. I might say, "Yeah, that's a great idea. Let's do that." Or they might say, "This person's on X dose of insulin. How 'bout we change it?" In that regard, I would use that nurse to help make suggestions and help make decisions. (Steve)

"Manage their care," "make sure that appropriate things are being done for them," "reinforcing their compliance and behavior," "help get this person under better control"—all things the primary care physician used to do and arguably is in the most legitimate position to still do personally. Things that arguably contain more of those interpersonal moments between doctor and patient that produce deeper knowledge of a patient's situation, lend greater voice to patients in the desire to have their doctor hear their story, and provide additional moments of social contact that produce a pool of experience for trust to take hold. Things that provide chances for each party to validate their belief in the other's ability to listen, dialogue, and show respect.

What many physicians interviewed didn't realize openly is that this work and in some cases, role transfer from doctor to non-physician staff person removed the physician further from what already had become, at least with respect to face-to-face doctor-patient interaction, an increasingly truncated affair—and one for which the patient already had lowered expectations. It limited doctor-patient touch points with patients, which, in turn, limited the total number of opportunities for physicians to exhibit relational features. Ironically, it was not a guarantee that any time saved for the doctor by shifting work to others produced greater face time between doctors and their patients, or more dyadic moments. In fact, even when talking about offloading work to others, most doctors did not see the move as solving their time-crunch problem. But what it did do was place others, not physicians, into situations where they were "caring for patients," even if at a more routine level. In all the primary care settings in which physicians were based, there was an emphasis on excelling at the transactional aspects of care, without the physician having to be involved.

The medical assistants are much more actively participating and managing, taking part in the patient's care, not just moving them from one room to another and taking their blood pressure. I think also, because they've [medical assistants] also kind of had that accountability and they're on the hook to drive those mammogram numbers and PAP smear numbers and those type of things, that when they're rooming those people, they're looking at their healthcare maintenance. They're asking about smoking status. They're checking if they're due for immunizations or labs. It's getting more and more automated. It's very rare that I order a mammogram anymore. Those are usually scheduled before I walk in the room. Similarly with colon cancer screening, oftentimes the conversation's already been had and the patient has a little home stool kit or else they have some questions for me about colonoscopies. If they're due for one, the MA starts that conversation. (Sid)

But what looked from the organization or physician's perspective like the rational use of a workflow innovation, namely, the use of a non-physician staff member to take over patient work, both the mundane and more complex, because of time, workload, or cost issues, nonetheless on another level created greater physical and psychological distance between physicians and their patients. This is even more apparent if one acknowledges, as physicians did in Chapter 4, that it was often during the seemingly "routine" interactions with patients that serendipity best manifested in the encounter, and when the opportunity for patients to talk, even about seemingly less relevant things, could reveal important clues for physicians to dig into further.

Some physicians were unapologetic in defending their use of non-physician staff members to interact with their patients and, by extension, to deliver some of their own meaningful relational value to them, even if they didn't have the M.D. initials after their names. They seemed to realize that most patients preferred interacting directly with them, but any guilt they felt in that regard was offset by a strong feeling of being put upon by their employers and the demands of the health care system. As a result, they tended to put the onus on patients for realizing and accepting this new reality, one they felt unable really to control or alter.

I think it's a big change for a lot of patients, and they don't understand why they don't just see their doctor in the 20-minute slots as they always have. Breaking them from that paradigm so that that dependence on the relationship with one physician is, I think, a challenge we've yet to really embrace and adjust well to. But it has to be done. Our reliance on that one to one, "I have my doctor, she's known me three years. That's the only person I see." That ultimately is going to be a hindrance, I think. We need to get them to understand, "These are my teammates, who are all equally invested in your care. We're going to meet together. You don't always have to see me. You might see my mid-level provider; you might see the pharmacist." Coach them [patients] on this model of care. We have a lot of work to do because people are a little bit weirded out by it. (Amy)

I wish patients knew that with this new model [team care using non-physician staff more in patient interactions], it's not just me and that person. I mean, it is when I'm in the room, but it's also my nurse practitioner. It's my medical assistant and whoever else has that contact with that patient. The patient expectation is still that you're their doctor and they're always gonna see you. That's just difficult to navigate in the present environment. (Pete)

PLACING FAITH IN THE PHYSICIAN'S ORGANIZATION, NOT THE PHYSICIAN

In the previous chapter, patients discussed their increasing view of the primary care physician as a "traffic cop," who, for example, gained them access to other parts of the system and steered them to the right specialists as needed.

I purchase the network of specialists that are within their [the primary care doctor's] system, and trust that they [the PCP] will get me into specialist appointments. She [the PCP] is really just a stepping stone. (Hallie)

This was presented as a lowered expectation on their part, that is, a belief based less in the doctor as someone with whom an ongoing relational experience could be had, and more as an instrumental asset for getting them [the patients] where they needed to go. This expectation of the primary care doctor as a "traffic cop" was accompanied by other feelings and opinions patients expressed that implied faith in the larger organizations of which many of their physicians were a part, either directly as salaried employees or indirectly through affiliations with hospitals or integrated delivery systems.

A number of patients were very comfortable with having their primary allegiances be to these larger organizations or systems of care. One widely noted reason for this comfort level was the belief that the larger organization could meet patient needs around convenience and assuring a form of quality control over accessing "good" doctors:

> That's actually another thing that I've come to really appreciate about that entire medical center. My primary care doctor is there. My OB/GYN is in that same building as well. I actually went to her because the PCP recommended her. The one that I ended up going with was the recommendation from her, and she's really fantastic. The whole practice is fantastic. But then they also have the lab there. They have an X-ray there, a whole bunch of things. It is kind of a one-stop shopping thing. It's very easy. (Lucy)

> What I like about the whole system is that everything is in the same building, the diagnostics and everything. Even the lab is there, everything. So it's convenient. (Krystal)

In addition, for patients with complex chronic diseases who accessed different doctors and parts of the system, and for healthy patients who were already in geographic proximity to a larger health care system, faith in the organization's "brand" also mattered. This faith was rooted in a feeling based less in relational trust and more in a sense of confidence in the public image or reputation of the organization. Some of these patients had ongoing experiences with their particular organizations, but the confidence expressed was not based on interpersonal interactions with specific doctors within those organizations, either primary care doctors or specialists. This feeling of "faith in brand" lessened patients' felt need to engage in complex decision-making about which specific doctors and organizations to go to for their care. In a situation where they felt fewer relational bonds with their primary care doctor, it was a short cut to simplifying the health care experience for themselves.

> As part of the organization, [ABC Health System], I get specialists, good ones. That's why I'm with them. That's why I'm not a free agent because I don't want to spend my time trying to figure out who I need to talk to. That's why this model works for me. It's because it cuts down my investment time. (Barry)

> I think I was comforted enough by—maybe it's just the aura of [XYZ Health System], but I was comforted enough knowing that these people knew what they were doing that you don't necessarily have to have the personal relationships develop there with any doctor. And I think it's kind of hard to develop those personal relationships if you're only seeing these people once or twice in a while. (Hadley)

> Living in that big city, [EFG health system] is obviously a big name there, and they have multiple hospitals all over the metro area, and as a result of that, they have multiple clinics, and so a reputable name. I went and checked it out, and ended up getting just randomly assigned to a [primary care] physician there. Even if my doctor left, I'd stay with the system, and just find another doctor there. (Edward)

In this way, patients gave a proverbial seal of approval to their physicians because of the larger organization to which they belonged, and not because they had a time-tested, deep pool of interpersonal experiences that showed off relational features consistently, or because that doctor knew them as unique individuals with particular life stories. Rather, because the larger organizations had already passed muster in their eyes, greater confidence was extended as well to the physician.

> I think that the quality level [of the system] is so high—it's a little idiot-proof in that way. I don't have to go and search three doctors

to find one that's good; I'm finding one good one pretty quickly. If they're going to be already—the things that I would look for— where they were trained and how long they've been doing the business, how many procedures they have, that type of thing— that bar has already been met by the fact that they're there [in the system]. So I don't have a problem with them [the primary care doctor] referring me within their system; it works more fluidly. The only value to this primary care doctor, why I wouldn't leave her is there's not a lot of them within this particular organization. And I have established what I think are pretty decent specialists within this system. Technically, I do like the fact that when my ENT guy is with me, he is able to access things that I have done elsewhere within the system if I tell him to. When I first moved here, I really wasn't sure what system I was going to be in. But this was a pretty dominant organization around here, well-known. (Hallie)

I certainly do think from time to time I would love to find a younger primary care physician who is, of course, understanding of men as we age, and I'd love that person to be at one of the major cancer hospitals in Boston. Most of my family members have over time moved their health care to be based at [ABC Health System] and to me that is a pretty impressive system. They seem to be doing some great things. (Matt)

Patients highlighted other ways in which they were giving themselves over to health care organizations rather than specific physicians. These included, as discussed earlier, a greater willingness to visit directly with non-physician providers such as nurse practitioners in some situations, especially those lower-level care instances where convenience and timely access were key interests. In concert with this expressed willingness to see non-physician providers was their comfort level with going to urgent care centers and retail clinics for primary care delivery; care delivery settings often owned and operated directly by large hospitals or corporations like CVSHealth, and which in many cases did not have physicians working in them on a regular basis.

These clinics you can literally just walk into. I do this when I'm out of town and something happens. But I've done that increasingly where I live over the last couple of years I think because I need something today. If there's something that I feel could wait till the morning, then I would probably call up my primary care physician and try and use that service. But if it happened at night or if it happened on the weekend, they're not available so I would go to these patient-first kind of places. (Hadley)

I usually go to urgent care over primary care but if I feel like it's something that just needs to be quick like I'm sick or something. (Tonya)

I'm very healthy, but if I am sick it's usually not at a convenient time for a primary care physician's office hours, something that would work for me, so having those options [retail clinics, urgent care centers] available I don't really feel that having a primary care physician is really that valuable actually. (Darlene)

The key facet to keep in mind here is that because these other care delivery options are often corporately owned and operated, for example, by hospitals, health systems, big box stores, or pharmacy chains, they already offer some of what the retail philosophy looks to sell. This includes pre-specifying through marketing messages a more limited array of standard medical services that can be delivered at a lower cost in some instances than at doctors' offices or emergency rooms. Retail clinics in particular embody the principles of scale, standardization, and price transparency employed through this philosophy. In addition, if one looks back at Table 1 in Chapter 3, it is clear that care delivery options such as urgent care centers and retail clinics are purely focused on maximizing transactional exchanges with patients. Visiting these organizations, short duration interactions are the norm. Patients may never see the same provider twice. There is no expectation of coming back for the same issue, creating distinct beginning and end points for the service transaction. Obligations between organization and patient are explicit (e.g., a set price for a specific diagnosis or service rendered). There is little to no continuity of care or development of ongoing relationships between doctor and patient (see Table 1, Chapter 3).

Thus, in their willingness to access care through these types of outlets, patients proactively engage in care delivery organized and administered through a retail lens, with an accompanying business model that looks upon physicians as high-cost labor inputs whose involvement in service delivery is less practical. This is not automatically negative in and of itself, given that it may lead to lower costs of care, although recent research shows that retail clinics are not the bastions of efficiency many presumed and may, in fact, increase health care spending (Ashwood et al. 2016). However, it connotes further drift between patients and doctors, particularly in the primary care sphere. Instead, an artificial bond arises between the organization and consumer, with the former interested in using their health care offerings as loss leaders that capture the latter as *buyers* of other services and products.

DISAPPEARING DOCTORS: WHAT IT MEANS FOR THE DOCTOR-PATIENT RELATIONSHIP

The increased reliance of patients and doctors on the larger health care organizations in which they are now embedded gives those organizations a close-in opportunity to connect with patients and develop their own version of relationships with them. In addition, given the level of resources and expertise needed, health care organizations and not individual physicians are in the strongest position to dictate the terms of how population health management and its tactics shape the delivery of medical care. For example, as we have heard, greater emphasis on care standardization, the use of metrics, and intense documenting and reporting requirements further eat up physician time, direct patients toward other non-physician staff, and marginalize direct interaction with patients. At the same time, patients begin to see value in allying themselves with the health care system rather than the individual physician, at the very least to have help in navigating services and doctors efficiently.

Working in combination, these realities help to "disappear" doctors in the eyes of patients, resulting in a gradual but steady diminishment of the physician's role as relational caregiver. This is not a small point. As the relational role diminishes, other perceptions gain fuel and feed back into a collective rationale for why a strong bond between doctors and patients is less needed and realistic. One perception is the belief among both primary care doctors and patients that the former's chief functions are to meet the demands of various organizational dictates through the rote administration of basic care management guidelines and clinical processes, justifying the "middleman" label described above. A second perception is that others on the health care team besides the doctor can and should provide relational care on a meaningful basis, raising the question of how much we need the already busy physician serving in such a role. Finally, as the relational role becomes a smaller part of the doctor-patient dyad, a self-fulfilling prophecy is created as both patient and doctor lose understanding and appreciation of this role, having fewer experiences of seeing it in action and realizing how meaningful it is. As mentioned in Chapter 4, this growing disappearance of physicians from the patient view occurs through physical and mental distancing, which makes it an insidious dynamic. Both occur when doctors knowingly or not cede more care responsibilities, decision-making, and control to the organization by adopting innovations such as checklist medicine or team care, which depend less on the substance of direct interactions between individual doctor and patient. For instance, greater use of health care teams in the delivery of care takes standard 15- or 20-minute office visits and further reduces the amount of that limited time a physician spends in front of a patient. Instead, medical assistants and nurses use significant portions of the visit at the outset and the end interacting with patients, helping to comply with quality requirements, and meeting the demands of checklist care. In some cases, as we have heard, these staff members know patients as well as the doctor does. Distancing also occurs when doctors overuse tools such as electronic health records that allow the organization to insert itself directly into the doctor-patient relationship within the exam room and beyond, directing how those interactions should play out, and influencing doctors to follow "scripts" that treat patients generically rather than uniquely.

The term "out of sight, out of mind" is applicable here. Psychologically, patients may begin to accept the reality that "seeing a physician," especially in primary care, is a rarer occurrence and something beyond their control to change. This belief facilitates the types of potential outcomes described at the end of the last chapter, including lowered expectations of doctors and gravitation toward new ways of interacting with the health care system. Health care organizations promote these new ways of interacting. For example, many primary care organizations have patients see a variety of providers over time, rather than a single physician, reducing the overall amount of contact time spent with one's "personal doctor." They do this because it's easier for scheduling and getting patients in the door, and often cheaper, but not because it is better for relational care delivery.

If significant parts of primary care work involve the use of detailed checklists and electronic record keeping to ensure that patients are "doing" the things required to stay healthy, the organization implicitly encourages physicians to further outsource interaction with their patients to lower-paid, less-trained personnel—who may work directly for the organization and not the physician. All of this leads to doctors knowing each of their patients less as individuals. And although health care teams can communicate to one another about specific patients through electronic health records, and physicians may believe they still know patients well through second-hand information gathered by others over disconnected points in time, relational features such as trust, empathy, and mutual respect between doctor and patient are less likely given such an asynchronous, indirect approach.

Mental distancing also occurs through how physicians working in roles such as "organizational middleman" and "traffic cop" come to think about their patients and their own personal capacity as professionals to provide relational care. The traffic cop role has been discussed already from the patient perspective, as patients' lowered expectations for primary care physicians (PCPs) interacts with the value they place on PCPs for getting them to "where they need to go," resulting in more patients who come to see their doctors for this purely instrumental reason. But the doctor's perspective is again worth noting here. Specifically, these two particular work roles (organizational middleman and traffic cop) are not likely able to make doctors satisfied in their jobs or careers. A recent survey of over 20,000 physicians nationally showed that much of why physicians felt the medical profession was in decline involved doctors having to absorb too much of the "middleman" role (because of excessive paperwork and regulation of their work), as well as the subsequent erosion of their relationships with patients (The Physicians Foundation 2014).

Rather, as heard in Chapter 4, doctors value the personal meaning found in performing relational care, and in their dyadic interactions with patients. Yet, these other roles, put upon them by employers, insurers, and accreditors, produce inner conflict for many physicians given the task- and process-oriented elements they contain and the time required for their fulfillment. This role conflict exacerbates the belief among many physicians that working as a paid employee of a hospital or larger organization such as an Accountable Care Organization or medical home does not help them provide better care quality or improve their relationships with patients (The Physicians Foundation 2014).

This inner conflict, alluded to in the Chapter 4 data and analysis, produces greater dissatisfaction and higher burnout among doctors in their work, and greater ambivalence or hostility toward some of their patients. Generally, individuals who do not understand the relevant features of a particular work role, or are asked to assume simultaneous incompatible work roles, are psychologically impacted in several ways, one of which involves the generation of negative feelings toward work, the job, and the career (House and Rizzo 1972). Both role ambiguity and role conflict in professionals can produce cognitive dissonance and uncertainty in knowing how to perform one's job effectively, helping to create these negative feelings (Piko 2006; House and Rizzo 1972).

It may well be that the current high levels of job dissatisfaction and burnout seen among primary care physicians, rates over 50 percent (see Shanafelt et al. 2015), are due in part to the tensions felt in attempting to enact their role as relational caregivers, while at the same time having to give significant attention to roles such as "traffic cop" and "middleman." Family physicians and general internists are at the top of the list when it comes to burnout and job dissatisfaction, and they are the doctors most involved in these organizationally driven roles (Shanafelt et al. 2015). Value discrepancy also comes into play here. To the extent there is a divergence felt by doctors between the value orientation of those paying them (e.g., insurers, employers such as hospitals) and their own value orientation, greater role stress results. This negatively impacts their perceived ability to provide the type of care delivery they want to their patients (Flaherty, Dahlstrom, and Skinner 1999). If doctors wish to provide relational care in their role as clinicians, but the organizations that pay them force too much of a focus on efficiency and moving patients through in a timely manner through standardized care delivery, because that is what *they* are most concerned about, some doctors will conclude that they cannot implement their preferred role with patients.

It is difficult for burned out or dissatisfied doctors to take the psychological risks needed to develop deeper relationships with patients, given what ends up being a reduced amount of internal motivation at their disposal (see Ryan and Deci 2000). As the central figure in their work, the patient in certain cases may become someone toward whom doctors feel guilty or resentful, especially if they unconsciously ascribe the blame for some of their negative feelings or role conflict to them. For instance, the noncompliant patient who complicates the role of organizational middleman may be someone from whom the physician mentally distances herself in an attempt to avoid further feelings of negativity. Dissatisfied or burned out doctors may, as a personal coping mechanism, carve these types of patients out of their everyday thinking, and be comfortable outsourcing interactions with them to other personnel, because to dwell on or engage with them simply brings more role stress. Ironically, such patients may need high doses of relational care (e.g., trust, empathy, dialogue) from physicians to change the way *they think* about their care. But they may become the ones least likely to get it.

On a simpler level, physicians may distance themselves psychologically from some patients because they do not like how those patients have come to view *them*. Given how the physicians in Chapter 4 discussed their views of the best, most meaningful doctor-patient relationships, it is safe to assume that being seen primarily as a "traffic cop" whose value for some patients lay in getting them "where they need to go" might make doctors feel disrespected or demoralized. They might ask themselves, "Why get to know or attempt relational care with such patients?" Interacting with patients who come through the door on a mission to go somewhere else may make doctors apprehensive about devoting emotional energy or time to relational care. Perhaps some primary care doctors embedded in the larger organizations in which patients exhibit confidence already know that they are not the deciding factor in why patients are with them. Such understanding could certainly lend itself to feelings of greater ambivalence toward select patients, perhaps *all* patients. This would be a normal human reaction to perceived slights from stakeholders (patients) whom they see as important to infusing meaning into their work and professional identity.

In the end, these negative psychological dynamics loom as significant destroyers of relational care potential in the doctor-patient dyad. They undermine the internal drive and explicit effort necessary for either party to cultivate bonds with each other. They lower the personal optimism required to enact relational features such as listening and empathy within everyday care contexts that are now hostile toward such things. They drain the available reservoirs of patience, trust, and goodwill that allow doctors and patients to give each other the benefit of the doubt when needed, and to wait longer for the payoffs from relational interaction. They help to estrange doctors and patients from each other, dumbing their relationship down into a series of discrete transactions that become highly strategic for serving the self-interest of one or the other party. They also offer greater opportunity for the health care organization to place itself in front of patients, which is discussed next.

WE'RE HERE FOR YOU NOW: REDEFINING THE "RELATIONSHIP" TOWARD ORGANIZATIONAL INTERESTS

As patient exposure to dyadic care with doctors—primary care or specialists— occupies a smaller percentage of their overall interactions with the health system, and as greater distance arises between the two groups, the medical profession has fewer real-time opportunities to serve as the legitimate stakeholder who defines the substance of the patient *experience*. There is much talk at present in health care about improving this experience, and overall recognition that it merits greater attention. First, it is embedded in the Institute of Medicine's quality mantra (Institute of Medicine 2001), making it a legitimate focus for the health care industry.

As such, it is measured through surveys like CAHPS (discussed earlier) and has been linked in meaningful ways to health care payments (Centers for Medicare and Medicaid Services 2016). Health industry executives have cited the patient experience as a key focus for their organizations to improve upon (Beryl Institute 2017), and highly paid consultants are available to help everyone from hospitals to physicians' offices grasp the concept and strategize around it.

"Patient experience" has become one of the key industry buzz terms of this decade. As a concept, however, it is all over the map at the present time. It has no clear definition or thought leader, meaning that different stakeholders in the industry think of it in different ways, and develop a variety of strategies for addressing it that span all parts of the business. To some it is more about the substance of the clinical interaction, that is, how well a patient's disease is cared for and treated. To others, it also means the nonclinical aspects of service delivery, that is, things such as wait times, whether or not patient parking is free, if there is a Starbucks or Panera Bread close by, and if there are online capabilities that patients can use to make appointments and see their test results in convenient ways. For the health care organization or system, it likely means all of these things and more.

Given the ongoing ceding of care to the corporation, and the gradual disappearance of the physician both physically and psychologically from the patient's view, the fact that the term "patient experience" has no clear consensus plays to the organization's advantage in defining it in ways that align with retail thinking. Specifically, health care organizations may tie the concept closer to the notion of seeing patients more as "consumers," that is, as entities with whom the organization can connect in different ways, all with the idea of building stronger *buyer–seller relationships*. Such relationships, as Chapter 5 points out, are less interpersonal and more transactional; less relational and more instrumental (i.e., targeted to fulfilling the narrow needs of particular customer segments); and use brand to build and sustain customer loyalty.

What is particularly important to appreciate is that the ceding of care to the corporation allows health care organizations to put themselves before individual patients more frequently in a variety of ways, which is a key success factor for engaging customers through retail approaches that require diverse "touch points" to build lasting brand and positive trans-actional experiences. Among other advantages, this gives the organization the strongest chance of defining what a "good experience" is for the patient; and that definition will take many forms. As noted earlier and in the previous chapter, patients may not be fully aware that this transitioning of the chief "experience" driver from doctor to organization is occurring. But this dynamic could further encourage the decline of physician influence in shaping patient care.

Even a role like "traffic cop," which may impact the doctor-patient relationship negatively but still give the doctor some degree of credibility and meaning in the patient's eyes, can slowly be taken away from primary care physicians, as their employing organizations use technology, big data, and other personnel to perform this role directly for patients. For example, although a patient's personal physician working within a larger system may have some firsthand knowledge of which specialists within that system are best to recommend for a given patient, or can perhaps make a call to get the patient in quicker to see someone in that system, there is little reason at this point that the larger organization cannot do these sorts of things equally well, perhaps even better than the physician. This is especially true the more doctors become salaried employees or independent contractors, floating around jobs and organizations in ways that do not allow them to develop their own relationships with specialists, which would give them the necessary tacit knowledge to guide patients.

In addition, the organization can provide the patient with many different types of information, beyond the limited information doctors can provide, to help them make informed decisions about whom to see and why, where in the system to access and how. For example, they can provide clinical performance information and rate doctors against one another. In addition, the organization can directly control scheduling for visits with specialists in ways that allow it and not the physician to be the sole arbiter of when patients are seen and whom they get to see. In these ways, much of the traffic cop role for physicians working in larger organizations is reduced simply because having the organization do it is more efficient, especially if an overriding goal is to coordinate timely access for large numbers of patients who need similar doctors and services.

For the organization, closer proximity to patients opens the door for greater opportunity to try new things with them; make service delivery or product innovation mistakes and recover from these without hurting their brand or reputation; and have a large customer audience with whom to do business. It creates the sort of mutual interdependency off which the retail philosophy feeds, with patients relying on the organization to help them make sense of a complex array of services, and the organization needing patients to transact with them on a scale that allows adequate profit margins and growth in market share. It lets the organization gain access to lots of "big data" in the form of personal and medical information, a critical ingredient to being a retail power, enabling the building of huge repositories that the organization uses for pushing out new services and products. It allows patients to believe that they have greater product variety at their disposal.

But as described in Chapter 3, this mutual interdependency, if defined by retail thinking, is not inherently geared toward achieving equity, fairness, or social justice—three things many believe go into a highly functioning health care system. It is not intended to establish or support deeply trusting emotional connections between individual doctors and their patients. By its nature, it does not promote empathetic or compassionate behavior. Rather, it is geared to creating "demand" and "selling things," not all of it health care related, to patients. It transforms the idea of "relationship" into a *monetized* one, where streams of stable, profitable (to the organization) transactions become the underlying logic driving how service delivery is structured (Booz and Co. 2008). Through the retail lens, organizations treat patients as "rational consumers" weighing the pros and cons of one health care purchasing decision over another (Volpp et al. 2011), while trying to convince them that certain purchases are worth more than others in terms of meeting their needs, wants, or preferences (i.e., things the organization also seeks to shape). Ideally, patients become informed and engaged, able to make these decisions in intelligent ways.

Health care organizations will have us believe that everyone wins in the end, and that the story is a familiar one, much like those seen in other sectors where a company like Amazon, Walmart, or Apple becomes highly successful and revered because it puts "the customer" first in considering how it conducts business, with the focus placed on appealing words such as "value," "timeliness," "convenience," "innovation," and "choice." Who wouldn't want more of these types of things in health care, an industry that for the better part of its existence has shown many failings, all of which impact us as patients in potentially adverse ways? The ongoing ceding of care to the corporation, of the kind alluded to in this chapter, sets the stage for a new narrative to take hold in health care, one that many believe holds much promise for not only meeting The Triple Aim, but also for modernizing our delivery system to fall in line with other segments of the economy that to many know how to engage consumers and satisfy them.

But here's the problem. At this point, it is shaping up to be an either–or proposition. We cannot know whether the two ways of thinking about health care delivery—dyadic, relational care typified by doctor-patient bonds versus population-based, transactional care that feeds into the application of retail thinking—are compatible in any meaningful sense right now. This is because the contextual backdrop in which they are embedded heavily promotes the pursuit of the latter at the direct expense of the former. As we have heard here, strong relational care between doctors and their patients is seriously threatened and, if these voices are to be believed, heading toward a no-turning-back transformation into something greatly reduced and different. Still, the voices here tell us, as well as the empirical research and our own common sense, that strong doctor-patient relationships of a dyadic nature have much value, and when operationalized in true fashion through the features identified fulfill both parties in ways that make the delivery of health care more humane, relevant, personally satisfying, and of higher quality. How to attempt to preserve and grow these relationships, lift the expectations of both doctors and patients, and restore greater humanity within the health care system, is the subject of the last chapter.

Chapter 7

Saving the
Doctor-Patient Relationship
and Raising Expectations

This point bears repeating: We are moving quickly toward a corporately controlled, transactionally focused health care delivery system, one that sees patients as "consumers" and doctors as high-cost, difficult to control labor. For doctors or anyone else to expect that we can go back to the days when medical care was delivered through smallish "mom-and-pop" physician-controlled practices, which used the hospital and other health care organizations at their leisure, is akin to believing in the early 1900s that horse travel would ultimately once again reign supreme, even as Model T's rolled off the assembly line. It is not realistic. There was no single tipping point, no precise day and time when it happened. Instead, as discussed in the early part of this book, it has played out over several decades through myriad strategies and tactics used to "improve" care quality, provide "better access" to services, and make health care delivery "more efficient" and "transparent." These strategies and tactics also have been used to reign in physician discretion over the work of patient care.

There have been many good intentions. The reality is, however, that accompanying all of it has been (a) the rise of a large corporate apparatus within health care organizations to handle the increased "complexity" of delivering and getting paid for care; (b) the retreat of doctors into salaried employment and toward the practice of medicine as a "job"; (c) the transfer of key physician roles to the organization, fracturing physician connections to patients; and (d) the implementation of technologies such as electronic health records, which allow the monitoring, quantification, and standardization of physician work, placing the organization into a more powerful position vis-à-vis patients. Regardless of what happens to the Affordable Care Act, what replaces it, or which political party is in power, these types of changes will continue to move forward, because they are a function of the ascendance of a larger market-based view on how service industries should function. That view is bipartisan.

What we have learned from hearing the voices of doctors and patients, embedded within this changed context of health care delivery is that the doctor-patient relationship faces a long and difficult road in gaining back a good measure of the influence it once had in our health care system. In fact, such heavy influence is likely gone for good. The relationship and its traditional focus on dyadic care delivery and the doctor as focal point for every patient encounter is not well aligned with the retail-oriented philosophy many in the business see as a next best way to advance their own interests under the guise of meeting multiple imperatives in such areas as care quality, efficiency, and population health.

Health care must and will continue to evolve, this advancing narrative goes, and that evolution can create new types of relationships between health care *buyers* and *sellers*, turn patients into *engaged consumers*, and let organizations, which have the proper scale and resources, fulfill a range of promises to patients on which physicians could never make good. Health care services will be treated more like *commodities* and a supportive *marketplace* will surround patients to empower and give them informed choices. The new health care relationships will consist of shorter-term, discrete transactions strung together over time in highly reliable and explicit ways to create a better buying experience overall. Everything will be more transparent, reliable, responsive, and consistent. Neglected goals, including convenience, timely access to needed services, and "getting people where they need to go" will be pursued seriously; and innovations in the industry will orient toward meeting those goals. Physicians will still play an important role, but so will other health care workers and technological innovations that deliver care at lower cost, and that will be fine. That's the story retail-favoring voices want us to believe.

At that level of abstract rhetoric, who can argue? For many, a physician-centric delivery system, particularly in primary care, has been too expensive, too difficult to control and make efficient, and too out of step with the sorts of disruptive innovations that are waiting (according to the emerging narrative) to make our health care lives better. In addition, as we have heard, it is not all that clear anymore how much doctors and their patients engage in deep, trusting relationships on a regular basis. For the naysayers, using interpersonal and dyadic relationships, especially with physicians, as the core foundation for the delivery of health care services no longer works given physician shortages, the large numbers of insured individuals, continued system fragmentation, new tools at our disposal, and the unnecessary service variation such dyadic relationships produce.

Thus, armed with a perception that it "is in the right place at the right time"; a confident marketing message with practical appeal; and a belief that it may not be undermining all that much between doctors and patients, the retail narrative moves as a powerful undercurrent through the myriad changes sweeping through the system at the present time. It justifies care standardization, quantifying doctors' work, and oversimplifying what goes into "good care delivery" through its myopic attention to process and "value." Within it, health care quality leans heavily toward a "conformance to specifications" endeavor, something little different in nature than assessing the quality of a Toyota coming off the assembly line, one after another. The retail narrative moves health workforce change in directions that use less-skilled labor to lower the marginal costs of delivering care and increase the profit margins of single health care transactions involving patients. Perhaps most important, the retail narrative promotes a view of the health care delivery setting as a "messed up" place requiring extended management interventions that include the use of scientific management techniques and electronic medical records. In this way, improving "workflow" and decreasing "waste" gain traction instead of ensuring that meaningful relational care consisting of emotional and psychological bonding is maintained between doctor and patients.

The problem is that the retail narrative and the actions it promotes within the system remain largely unproven, and anathema to the moral justifications for why we want a strong doctor-patient relationship at the center of health care delivery. Maybe the types of strong, effective doctor-patient relationships described in this study are not all that common anymore, if they ever were before. But in a key sense it doesn't matter. After all, health care is an area of our lives where at key junctures we want to *believe* in the relational side of things, specifically, that trained individuals care about what happens to us, and use their expertise to try and help improve our lives, and the lives of our friends and families. We want to have the basis for hope in such a system, even if it is not fully realized.

Retail thinking and its view of the patient as a "consumer" is not consistent with this view of care delivery as an inherently *humane* endeavor. Patients are not Toyotas, they are unique individuals with particular life stories, circumstances, and needs—all of which shape who they are as healthy or unhealthy individuals. Ironically, retail thinking applied to health care has less evidence and a smaller cadre of positive experiences over time associated with it than the narrative of how and why strong doctor-patient relationships matter. Still, these market-oriented ideas rush in to fill a void left by the slow degradation of the relational ideal. In its defense, the retail narrative is not responsible for destroying that relationship as much as taking advantage now of its demise. It is an opportunistic set of strategies and tactics, driven in part by corporate profit seekers from both inside and outside the industry, as well as big organizations that want to grow and gain market share.

What the retail narrative is directly responsible for, however, is letting many unproven assumptions about doctors and patients undermine the case for maintaining strong relational bonds between doctor and patient. *Physicians never were all that connected to their patients in the first place. Physicians cannot be trusted to provide the right kind of care to their patients. Patients want more now than a strong relationship with their doctor. Patients want to control their health care decision-making. Dyadic care between doctor and patient is wasteful and inefficient, and too misaligned with the complexities of today's health system. Patients love technology in their health care. The health care organization is in a better position to provide a more robust patient experience. Features such as interpersonal trust are impossible to quantify in terms of their benefit for health care outcomes. Treating patients at a population level makes more sense than treating them as unique individuals. Variation in service delivery is a bad thing, indicating a wasteful doctor. Technology can solve the ills of the delivery system by lowering costs and giving patients more control.*

This list of assumptions goes on, promulgated in ways designed to convince us that we can have something better, something less complicated and cheaper. It seeks to have us believe that perhaps we do not have to rely on those busy and expensive physicians we cannot seem to ever get in front of us but instead turn ourselves over to the reliability of large health care organizations. The view taken in this last chapter is that it's not fine to swallow these types of assumptions blindly, in part because most of them have little truth. There is no good reason to downplay the doctor-patient relationship, especially in the area of primary care service delivery. Serious reservations emerge from considering a health care system in which that person-to-person relationship is left to wither on the vine, replaced by something much more impersonal and market-driven.

But certain realities are here to stay. Thus, any discussion of how to keep the doctor-patient relationship vibrant and meaningful must pay heed. Metric fever in health care is not going away and, if anything, will continue to establish itself as the new normal across all of health care delivery. This will be the case whether the Affordable Care Act is the law of the land or something else replaces it. There will be fewer primary care physicians in the future, at least not as many as needed to keep up with patient demand, and shortages of many different types of doctors likely will exist in the United States (Association of American Medical Colleges 2016; Hoff and Pohl 2017). To provide the greatest number of patients with reasonable access to care increasingly will mean greater use of non-physician providers, health care teams, and technology that reduces the need for face-to-face visits and pushes patients to manage themselves.

The time squeeze doctors face in their workday will continue to mean shorter visits for all patients, impacting the ability to engage in relational care (Rabin 2014). Doctors often adjust to less time with patients by becoming more directive in their interactions, letting the patient talk less, and interrupting them more (Hoff 2010; Langewitz et al. 2002). The heavy workloads doctors also face may make many of them turn away from the hard road of developing deeper relationships with their patients, and instead focus them even more on getting through their workdays efficiently, getting home on time, and emphasizing the nonwork pursuits in their lives (Caryn 2014; Hoff and Pohl 2017).

Relatedly, doctors will continue to become salaried employees and independent contractors in greater numbers. As they settle in as paycheck workers in models such as patient-centered medical homes and accountable care organizations, working for larger corporate organizations and systems, they will continue to transfer traditional roles to their employers; roles that in toto enhance their value in the eyes of patients and add to their ability to develop good relationships with patients. This role transfer and the capturing of physicians as wage workers shifts power and influence to the health care organization, which will continue to argue that it is in the best position (as opposed to individual doctors) to serve patients across an array of various needs and preferences. Patients, increasingly befuddled by a world of excessive insurance plan variety, greater out-of-pocket expenses, restrictive choices regarding which physicians they can see, and a delivery system still highly fragmented will place more faith in the health care organization to help them make sense of it all.

Finally, the philosophy and tools of population health management (PHM) should remain ascendant in American health care delivery, in part because the fuel that drives the PHM engine remains a mix of future technologies and capabilities that the industry (and venture capital coming into health care) has bought into, such as the use of "big data," artificial intelligence, and algorithm-driven care. For example, there is great enthusiasm for using technology like IBM's Watson supercomputer to diagnose and treat patients (IBM 2016), and for using web- and app-based tools such as symptom checkers that can allow patients to self-diagnose without needing to visit a doctor. Technology companies like Apple seem poised to assume a greater role in health care delivery (Bryant 2016). The era of "cognitive health" is upon us, and a significant part of that era will be defined by the use of machine learning, powerful computer algorithms, and cloud computing to manipulate and store troves of patient data for segmenting patient subpopulations. At its conceptual best, PHM offers the system order and efficiency in terms of how standardized care can be delivered based on the more homogenous needs of patient groups.

The remainder of this last chapter does not offer magic bullets or fantastical propositions for preserving relational care between doctor and patient in our health care system. It would be irresponsible and against the empirical proof offered in this book to do so. It tries, however, to outline at a strategic level several ways the system can become more ready, willing, and able to engage doctor-patient relationships and relational care in more meaningful ways. It provides some tactical suggestions for raising doctor and patient expectations related to interactions with each other. It is an uphill battle, however, and everything discussed keeps the realities outlined in this study in mind at all times, acknowledging that the doctor-patient relationship moving forward within the American health care system is forever hamstrung by an unfavorable context in which to prosper.

BECOMING MORE READY: THE MEDICAL PROFESSION'S NEED TO DRIVE AND FOCUS ON RELATIONAL CARE

I have worked with and studied doctors for three decades and have learned a lot about them during that time. I am also a trained professional myself. Given this, I have a keen appreciation for the particular mindsets doctors employ; the defensive routines that typify their aversion to change; and the way in which they construct their various identities as service providers and workers, in large part because I probably think and respond to my world in much the same ways they do. From my 2010 book on the work of primary care according to the doctors living it, I came away with the conclusion that primary care physicians were giving up too much in terms of complex work, decision-making autonomy, and direct contact with their patients, in their minds for strategic reasons and to make ends meet within a delivery system that was shortchanging their work and questioning their value. However, these actions also helped to fracture their relationships with patients long-term, and this is what many of them did not seem to understand.

As we have seen in this book, what primary care physicians now give up to improve their economic situations, lifestyles, and ability to navigate busy workdays are in fact key roles and work that has a direct impact on what patients think of them and their ability to build and maintain relationships with those patients; for example, jettisoning care for their patients in the hospital; shifting basic but foundational patient contact (e.g., taking vital signs and performing some of the standard yet "getting to know the patient" physical and history data collection) to non-physician staff; keeping visits shorter and more directive in terms of the conversations had with patients; referring patients out too quickly to specialists, and turning medicine into a nine-to-five job that conveys to patients that their needs are not important. These things clearly feed into the lowered expectations patients now have of them, described here in detail, and into their own inability to grow and sustain important features of relational care (e.g., trust) on an individual basis (see Hoff 2010). It also has reduced physicians' opportunities to have extended relational moments with their patients, and in the process decreases their "on the job" training exposure to developing key relational skills.

In this study, though, we see how much dyadic care and emotional bonding with patients still resonates with primary care doctors, which makes the reality all the more disheartening. It gives tremendous meaning to their work and careers. Its absence is a source of burnout and cynicism. It feeds into the creation of a satisfying professional identity. It motivates them. We heard how much physicians value those everyday experiences in which there are high relational moments of interaction, that is, where features such as trust, listening, empathy, and dialogue are in great abundance, and where they can play a variety of roles, including friend and confidante, which bring them emotionally and psychologically closer to their patients. But we also see physicians who feel increasingly disempowered to change things, whose lessening chances to practice relational care, and whose own involvement in ceding roles to the corporation, cause them to distance themselves psychologically from their patients.

Into this paradox emerges two clear messages for doctors, particularly those in the field of primary care—first, *start caring more about building strong relationships with your patients and, second, start preparing yourselves better, even within hostile work contexts, to nurture and maintain the kinds of patient relationships you already know are vital to good health care, satisfied patients, and your own job and career satisfaction.* Advance preparation for strong relationship building matters more now than ever, in large part because doctors face a delivery system that will discourage them at every turn from bonding with their patients in ways that build trust and emotional connections. Knowing ahead of time how and why such relationships matter for themselves and their patients, and being able to engage in requisite features such as empathy, compassion, and listening—in ways that are efficient and do not require highly favorable conditions—raises the chance that tomorrow's doctors can achieve some success in maintaining bonds with their patients. It may never be what it once was or what doctors thought it once was, but it can still be meaningful.

At present, it would be incorrect to say that doctors collectively are properly readied through their training and work experiences to practice relational care generally, and certainly not within the type of corporatized delivery system this book has described. Medical schools and residency programs have failed students and residents in this regard, by not letting them see in full glory the mutually rewarding essence of relational care, and by not equipping them with the capabilities, personal resilience, and mindsets with which to pursue it. In many ways, the early preparation of doctors, from the start of medical school through the end of residency, remains fixated on developing technical competence and absorbing impersonal scientific facts at the expense of developing relational care capabilities. The emphasis is on book smarts rather than emotional intelligence; on individual organ systems and body parts rather than whole people and life histories.

With few exceptions, medical schools and residency programs still do not fill the doctor's toolbox with the kinds of thinking, skills, and emotional maturity needed for developing and maintaining strong patient relationships. As a result, once dropped into a highly transactional delivery system where time is of the essence and standardized performance measures are everywhere, many of these young physicians choose the paths of least resistance, one of which is simply to see their patients as efficiently as possible, perhaps get to know some a little and others not at all, comply with the metrics placed on their work, and perform their jobs in ways that are seen as technically competent. All the while turning as much as possible over to the employing organization, and focusing on trying to be a master of the electronic medical record rather than of the patient experience.

The harmful effects such ambivalence for relational care has on young doctors is palpable. For example, one recent review of 18 separate studies showed that medical trainee empathy actually decreases during medical school and residency (Neumann et al. 2011), despite other evidence showing that even minor additional teaching in that particular skill improves patients' perceptions that the medical trainee is practicing empathetic care (Riess et al. 2012). Reasons cited for the decline of empathy among trainees include the intense workloads and student burnout associated with medical school and residency, as well as fewer bedside interactions and a lack of care continuity with the same patients over time, as students move through clerkships and then engage in residencies within settings such as hospital clinics that function more as safety net providers than continuous care settings (Neumann et al. 2011).

The lack of patient continuity in medical student and resident training experiences is a significant barrier to improving young physicians' capacity to perform relational care. Dynamics such as trust are interpersonal and longitudinal. They manifest best through extended contact between doctor and patient, and the development of a shared pool of positive interpersonal experiences. One solution offered to this problem is that of the longitudinal clerkship, which supports having physician trainees work with the same patients over time, in part to cultivate relationships with them and see how their work is shaped by knowing the patient and their circumstances (Dow and Reeves 2016). As Dow and Reeves (2016, p. 161) note, immersing trainees in continuous care with the same patients while learning how to become doctors enables opportunities for them to hone (and see the firsthand importance) of skills such as empathy and trust. By seeing the favorable impact of these skills on patient care and how positively patients respond to this type of care, young doctors are more likely to enter into full-time practice committed to using these skills in the regular course of their work.

Despite talk of recent Medical College Admission Test (MCAT) revisions that focus more on identifying students who may possess good relational skills as future doctors, the reality is that most medical schools and residency programs underemphasize student exposure to relational medicine (Schwartzein 2015). It's fine to bring more students in who have relational care potential, but if one then puts them through training that underwhelms on the relational front, all one is doing is creating an even larger pool of dissatisfied doctors down the road. Admitting more students to medical school who possess greater potential for building strong relational skill sets compared with others means little unless those same schools inject every aspect of their curriculum with a pedagogic focus on how to build and maintain strong doctor-patient relationships. In short, one needs a significant dose of nurture to complement the nature of student selection. In this way, wholesale revisiting of the medical school curriculum and residency experience to critically assess how each part of both does or does not train students to excel at relational care should be a strategic imperative of oversight organizations such as the Association of American Medical Colleges (AAMC) and the Accreditation Council on Graduate Medical Education (ACGME).

Improving medical training and residency experiences around relational care is not the only imperative for the medical profession. There is also a practice imperative. As this book describes, for doctors in the field, their relationships with patients are threatened with what have become normalized ways of contracting for their labor, organizing and monitoring their work, and paying them. On many fronts of everyday practice, physicians are losing their ability to put in place circumstances that favor the plying of their relational trade on a dyadic level. As a result, there is an increasing need for practicing physicians to bargain collectively for the kinds of working conditions (e.g., patient care schedules, job structures) that at their worst will not undermine the physician time, motivation, and capacity needed to perform relational care, and at their best offer a more supportive context for physicians to cultivate and strengthen deeper patient relationships. As more doctors become salaried employees, their everyday working conditions, rather than insurance reimbursements (given that most are paid a salary) become the key focal point for improvement.

Traditionally, the profession as a whole, particularly in primary care, has fought and bargained over reimbursement. That singular focus continues today. For example, primary care physicians went all in recently on participating in "patient-centered medical homes," but not because they believed it would provide a better work context in which to engage relationally with patients. Rather, most also thought it would bring additional resources and reimbursement that could alleviate the strains their practices were feeling. That it has not produced a financial windfall, but actually required additional resource investment to meet the quality improvement demands of the various checklists that convey to accreditors and insurers that they are "medical home certified," has added to physician cynicism that relational care is not possible on a grand scale.

Currently, an enormous amount of physician energy is spent on pushing back against Medicare and private insurers to shape how reimbursement evolves in the health care delivery market. This constant fight over dollars to the detriment of other elements of physician practice supports the idea that the American medical profession remains too preoccupied with its own economic status rather than its cultural legitimacy with individual patients. By over focusing on reimbursement at the expense of things like working conditions and the quality of patient relationships, the profession misses the mark in preserving its' members capacity to provide relational care to patients. As Starr (1982) and Abbott (1988) pointed out decades ago, physicians' economic status is a direct function of their cultural legitimacy, which gives them the ascendant position of chief authority in health care. Cultural legitimacy, in turn, is partially dependent upon how patients see and experience doctors as a key source of relational care. As we heard from patients, physicians as professionals decrease in stature and relevance to some patients when the relational experience pool is shallow. This opens these patients up to seeing the organization or perhaps other health care workers as legitimate sources for their care which, over time, may shift allegiances toward the corporation.

Whether or not physician labor unions are the future for this type of collective bargaining (see American Academy of Family Physicians 2016; Scheiber 2016), or whether traditional professional trade groups like the American Medical Association or state-level associations can unite physicians to negotiate better workplace conditions, there is little doubt this focus will become imperative (Page 2016). As physicians increasingly are salaried or contractual employees, subject to "at will" employment arrangements that depend in part on how much their performance complies with organizational mandates around quality and efficiency, the need to unite locally amongst themselves and perhaps with others such as nurses makes sense (Union of American Physicians and Dentists 2016). Although existing labor laws always loom as an obstacle to collective bargaining for doctors when they are presumed to be "supervisors" as well as clinicians, many of them now fit the definition of "employee" that is consonant with gaining collective bargaining status (Leffell 2013).

Organized medicine must first formally recognize how certain work and employment conditions, particularly those associated with metric fever, care standardization, and value-based reimbursement negatively impact their members' ability to do their jobs in the manner they prefer, a big part of which is providing relational care. The profession must understand how patient care expectations toward doctors shift in the context of these circumstances. In this study, doctors spoke of needing time to listen and ask patients' questions about their lives; of conveying an air of accessibility and accountability to patients; and of being able to see the same patient over time to develop the shared experiences that produce interpersonal trust and tacit knowledge of individual circumstances. How is all this possible without doctors pushing back against their employers and the larger system in relation to the constraints now placed upon their time and work? How do conditions on the ground change with the most powerful worker in the system, the one still possessing the most credibility with customers, essentially sitting on the sidelines and not pushing proactively against the rising tide of workflow redesign, efficiency experts, and transactional medicine that others think holds the answer to a better health care system?

Physicians must articulate and pursue a clear action agenda for improving those working conditions that occupy the top of their negotiating wish lists, both locally and on a national basis. Negotiating work conditions with their employers is not something that physicians initially may feel comfortable about doing or be all that good at, given their own professional beliefs that such a focus is beneath them. Yet, there must be a realization on their part that what they like most about their jobs is directly threatened by some of the surrounding features of everyday practice. They must finally recognize that they are indeed "workers" whose ability to control their daily fates has been reduced greatly (Hoff 2001). They must acknowledge collectively the threat from corporate organizations bent on reducing their high-cost presence across as many care delivery workflows as possible, whether through the use of team care, artificial intelligence, electronic medical records, or smartphone apps.

Physicians collectively must warm to the idea that most of them no longer control all the terms of their working arrangements, having bartered meaningful portions of that power away to their employing organizations in exchange for better lifestyle considerations or short-term insulation from the business pressures of making ends meet. As a result, much as early unionized workers fought for an eight-hour workday, and nurses bargain for more supportive conditions in which to care for their patients, physicians will want to collectively bargain for things like minimum standard face-time allotments with patients who visit them in the office each day. They will want to negotiate with their employers for caps on the total number of patients they are required to see in a given daily work schedule, the overall size of their patient panels, and the specific requirements for using the electronic health record during or after patient visits. These types of things directly affect their ability to develop ongoing relationships with the same patients over time, and to listen, dialogue, show compassion, and engender trust.

There surely is reluctance for the American medical profession to embrace a view of their members, particularly early-career doctors, as put-upon workers struggling to gain favorable conditions for their work within corporatized health care settings. But that view already has been borne out by the facts on the ground; by the willingness of the profession to engage vigorously in fights over cuts and modifications to physician reimbursement in all its forms; and in survey after survey of doctors showing high job dissatisfaction, high burnout, and excessive administrative workloads. The prestige of doctors is not negatively impacted by continually waking up to the fact that their work is now highly dictated to them through performance metrics, organizational policies, and outcome-focused payment schemes. After all, the prestige of the medical profession in a country like England remains high, even as the British Medical Association supports its junior doctors going on strike to gain better working conditions (Triggle 2016). What it takes is clear, pragmatic thinking by the profession in understanding what is happening to doctors in the trenches, and the institutional bravery to take risks with the general public in showing these professionals as increasingly beholden to the growing power and control of health care organizations.

Being More Willing: Convincing Organizations and the Marketplace to Want Relational Care

In a health care system trending toward greater consumerism and retail thinking, the future viability of relational care between doctor and patient in part hinges on the ability to create an additional set of value propositions around such care that resonates with the idea of patients as "customers"; with the health care organizations that increasingly employ physicians; and with business interests in the larger marketplace. To some, this point may seem both contradictory and distasteful, especially given the analysis above about physicians collectively bargaining for better working conditions and the acknowledgment that relational features such as trust, empathy, dialogue, and compassion are realized most fully through ongoing, interpersonal exchanges between people, and not through care delivery that overemphasizes transactional qualities such as speed and convenience. As threaded throughout this book, there is much about retail thinking that is anathema to effective relational care delivery occurring between doctor and patient.

But realities are realities. The American health care system is embracing a future in which the overall physician role, particularly in primary care, likely continues to diminish; regular direct face time with primary care physicians grows harder to achieve for every patient; patients identify more with the health care system for helping them make decisions and navigate their care (in part because their insurance plans make them do it this way); and new technologies and innovations continue to disrupt the doctor-patient connection. In addition, there simply are not enough doctors in parts of medicine like primary care to satisfy the goal of dyadic relationships that deliver on the relational promise for each and every patient. The support of the health care corporation, with its resources and coordinating power, must be enlisted to help if the doctor-patient relationship has any meaningful chance at flourishing in the years ahead, and doing so for the largest number of patients in the system. But it may have to look somewhat different and involve heavy doses of virtual contact between doctor and patient.

In a market-oriented delivery system, the physician's preeminence in maintaining direct interpersonal relationships with patients that deliver on things like trust may be preserved to some degree if that type of relationship is recognized not only for its ethical and moral values, or for its rich expression of humane caregiving, but also for its *business value*. Retail-oriented companies think transactional excellence first, but it does not preclude an interest in excelling at the human and interpersonal aspects of relational care if indeed their customers attach additional purchasing decisions to such things. By using the kinds of powerful data analytics now available, some health care organizations can, if relational care attributes are accurately measured (see the next section), find out for themselves if and how strong doctor-patient relationships feed into happier consumers who then extend this goodwill to thinking more positively toward the company's brand and, in the process, become better selling targets for the organization's full range of service and product offerings.

From the findings here, patients have increasingly lowered expectations that relational care is possible with their doctors. But it is also clear that they still need, want, and prefer such care when it is available. It has value for them. This qualitative information is bolstered by the existing array of research on the benefits of strong doctor-patient relationships, outlined in Chapter 1, and on data showing that regardless of how patients are segmented into different subgroups of "health care consumers," all of the various segments appear very interested in maintaining to some degree more traditional care approaches and interactions with their physicians (Deloitte 2012). To the health care organization, this knowledge is useful because it suggests there are viable value propositions for giving patients greater access to relational care that potentially not only benefit patient care and physician well-being, but also enhance the company's image and bottom line.

As patients pay more directly out-of-pocket for the costs of care, some will come to make bigger demands as customers on how that care should look. Approximately 25 percent of all covered employees in the United States now participate in a consumer-directed health plan (CDHP), and more employers include such plans in their offerings each year (Mercer 2016). CDHP's are types of insurance plans that place greater financial accountability onto the patient through higher annual deductibles that must be met before services receive coverage, and higher copay amounts for certain services. The average out-of-pocket annual premium cost for a typical insurance plan with family coverage is approximately $5,000

(Kaiser/Health Research Educational Trust 2016). This figure, however, does not include consumers paying increasingly larger annual deductibles and an assortment of copays, especially if they have a CDHP. For many families, this adds several more thousand dollars annually to their out-of-pocket costs. The number of covered lives in CDHPs is expected to grow as employers continue to try and steer their workers toward such offerings to lower their own premium costs, and as individuals who purchase their own plans directly seek price discounts on the premium side in exchange for paying more to actually use the insurance.

It has long been argued that once they have "more skin in the game," individual patients will become engaged, astute purchasers of their care. This may be true to some extent. Perhaps one area where they could demand greater attention to their needs and preferences would be with respect to the amount of contact they wish to have with their physicians, and how they wish that contact to be structured. Some interviewees in this study were covered through CDHPs and did not necessarily express strong interest in having this type of input into their care. Several of them, however, were younger and did not need access to the system on a regular basis. Any "dormant" needs and preferences for relational care present within patients interviewed for this study could surface quicker if either the number of subpar interactions they have with the health care system increases or they pay more for their care.

Of course, good retail thinking is also about the organization that *sells things* being aggressive in "activating" consumers. In this way, health care organizations might facilitate a "push-pull" dynamic in the marketplace in which patient needs and preferences for relational care are given an expanding number of opportunities to be met, even if they all do not fulfill the ideal of dyadic, face-to-face interaction between doctor and patient. For example, could organizations that employ their physicians innovate in ways that raise patient expectations regarding relational care, and then provide additional products and services that supplement in positive ways the traditional dyadic relationship that is the foundation for such care?

For instance, perhaps a health care organization that already invests heavily in a state of the art electronic medical record system can find new ways to use that system to keep doctors and some of their patients in virtual touch with each other on a more frequent basis. Although we currently have electronic "patient portals" in many physician offices, the marketplace is still at a nascent stage of development in using such technology to bring doctors and their patients closer together. Most of the time, this type of technology works asynchronously and gets co-opted to perform the rote administrative chores of the practice, such as posting raw test results for patients to see, sending reminder letters from the practice, and communicating regarding billing issues.

Other ideas here could strengthen connections between doctors and their patients, although these are not without their concerns. Various social media sites like Facebook already are used by some medical offices to communicate with their patients, but the communication is primarily not patient-specific and instead is structured around advertising various services in the office (e.g., immunizations, flu shots), offering standard education around health issues for groups of patients, and conveying administrative information about the office. As younger generations weaned on this form of "weak tie" interaction grow older, such outlets could be used more to facilitate doctors and patients building relationships with each other. Making direct contact between the doctor and patient be the primary goal of using such technology could produce spinoff products that consumers might be willing to pay something extra for using in relation to their health care.

Perhaps there could be "concierge staff" within physician offices who are employed by the organization and work as direct liaisons between specific doctors and patients. These personnel would not function as such intermediaries (who are usually Medical Assistants or staff not trained in particular relational skills) do now, for example, running interference for the doctor with patients, or doing lower-level clinical tasks, but instead act as "communication" and "listening" relay stations that function as patient advocates first, and have as their chief goal to help build and maintain good connections between the two stakeholders. Perhaps other forms of technology such as smartphone apps, used at present to improve transactional excellence with respect to services like primary care (e.g., *ZocDoc, Doctor on Demand*), could be adopted by the organization as tools for increasing *relational excellence* between doctors and their patients, for example, by increasing knowledge flow back and forth between the two; providing a real-time outlet for patients to ask questions and be heard; and allowing the physician to respond quicker to patients and to seem more accountable.

One also could imagine some consumers being asked to pay extra, for example, for the right to see their doctors more in person or at a time convenient for them. In fact, we have a model like that now, called "concierge medicine," which at present exists on a small scale nationally and caters to affluent health care consumers willing to pay monthly or annual subscription fees for the right to have their personal doctor available at their leisure. The present form of concierge medicine is both expensive and difficult to scale up, given that individual physicians employing the model usually work as part of small offices, which can sign up only a limited number of patients to meet the goal of timely accessibility and strong relational care delivery. Costs for such a service, in addition to patients' insurance costs, can run into the thousands of dollars per year, and for most patients and doctors it is not feasible in its current form.

But what if the model could be made both more affordable and scalable? In fact, some large systems have begun trying to make the concierge medicine model a more legitimate part of their service offerings (Massachusetts General Hospital 2016). These larger organizations may be able to achieve certain efficiencies that allow them to sign up a larger group of patients for their doctors at a lower subscription price. Taking it one step further, to the extent the concierge model can be segmented to provide varying levels of physician accessibility and contact (e.g., "premium," "standard"), more patients may have at least some ability to participate in this type of care, which could better deliver on the relational promise. What has not been mentioned much are the prospects for other care providers, such as nurse practitioners (NPs) and physician assistants (PAs) to participate in concierge medicine. Given the shortages of doctors in primary care, using NPs and PAs as the relational focal point for some patients, particularly healthier ones, is a future reality that ironically furthers the de-emphasis on doctors already occurring in the system. At the same time, it allows patients the chance to bond with other skilled professionals who are helping them make decisions on their health.

These are small tactical suggestions. The larger imperative is to get the health care marketplace and organizational stakeholders within it to want to spend time, effort, and money on forging delivery contexts that bring doctors and their patients closer together. To see that happen, there is little doubt patients themselves also would need greater ability to vote with their feet, and move their business from one health system or organization to another when dissatisfied with the lack of relational care experienced. In this way, just as hotel chains like Marriott and Hilton, understanding that guests normally have plenty of lodging options when travelling, fixate on meeting customers' service preferences to enhance their brand, so, too, could hospitals and physician practices respond accordingly if they felt patients could not be taken for granted. Just paying more out-of-pocket for care will not activate consumers as smarter shoppers, or enable them to be in this power position. If most geographic regions end up with monopolistic or oligopolistic systems of care delivery, and health insurers continue to develop the concepts of "narrow networks" in which subscribers are given a limited number of participating hospitals and doctors to choose from, it is hard to see how relational care between doctor and patient gains economic value for the stakeholders involved.

BECOMING MORE ABLE: MEASURING AND INCENTIVIZING THE DELIVERY OF RELATIONAL CARE

We value what we measure. This statement reflects the opposite of an important business maxim. Nonetheless, it reflects the place of metrics in health care today. Metrics drive the industry's identification of areas to improve upon and reimburse. This will not change anytime soon. Too many powerful stakeholders believe that overquantification is better than worse for health care delivery. It is with such an understanding that a concerted effort should be made over the next decade to cultivate implementable, standardized measurements for relational features such as trust, empathy, respect, listening, emotional intelligence, and patient perceptions of both friendship and advising excellence with their doctors. Thom, Hall, and Pawlson (2004) note the importance of measurement with respect to trust, and it applies to all relational features:

> Measuring trust would also be an important complement to market forces. It could help focus market forces on sustaining or improving

trust as an aspect of health care quality. . . . every reason that exists
for measuring other aspects of quality applies with equal force to
measuring trust. Indeed, for some purposes, trust may be a more
encompassing and revealing measure than any of the others, either
alone or combined. (p. 128)

The Consumer Assessment of Health Plans (CAHPS) exists right
now as the most commonly used survey to tap into relational aspects of
patient care. But the selling of the CAHPS survey in its present form as
an appropriate tool to measure relational care is misguided. First, as mentioned earlier in the book, a few questions on a survey patients get after
a specific visit to a doctor's office does not tap into relationships. It taps
into the single visit transaction. Thus, nothing on the CAHPS clinician
survey right now is measuring how patients feel in or perceive their *ongoing relationship* with a doctor. Nothing is measuring their holistic experience interacting as a dyad with that professional. Second, the questions on
CAHPS that purport to assess relational care are incomplete, and maybe
don't measure relationship quality at all.

For example, they ask, "At your visit—Did your provider listen carefully to you?" "Did your provider explain things in easy to understand
terms?" "Did your provider show respect for what you had to say during your visit?" Are these questions better than nothing? Sure. But they
are wholly insufficient for assessing the full range of relational dynamics
occurring (or not) between an individual doctor and patient. They also
mislead in the sense that favorable responses (e.g., my provider did listen
to me during the visit!) are prone to overexaggeration by doctors and their
employers who then conclude that patients are getting good relational care
across the board, when, in fact, they are not. This misinterpretation can
lead doctors to make superficial rather than transformational changes to
improving the relational elements of their practice. Information gleaned
from these surveys also does not give them deep insights into how patient
expectations toward their care may or may not be changing.

In addition, these types of questions are more process-oriented, which
fits with metric fever's emphasis on making physicians *do certain things*
to or for patients, but runs counter to assessing accurately interpersonal
dynamics that are highly subjective (e.g., Do you *feel* like you trust your

physician to look out for you and make decisions that are in your best interest?) and whose most valid assessment comes through a combination of checklist-like process questions *and* more qualitative anecdote-sharing that can dive deeper into the full range of relational dynamics patients take away from interactions with their doctors. Add to that CAHP'S questions whose response categories are forced-choice rather than open-ended (Never! Sometimes! Usually! Always!), leaving little room for nuance. One can argue that such a tool as structured pays perhaps little more than lip service to wanting to know about the relational depth existing in dyadic doctor-patient relationships.

Although robust measures of an important relational feature like trust are scarce (Pearson and Raeke 2000), and would have to be developed and tested (see Thom, Hall, and Pawlson 2004), there are several well-rounded measures of a feature like empathy, which could be immediately used in standardized patient surveys such as CAHP'S (see Mercer et al. 2004). That said, measures of complex relational dynamics often merit more than single questions on surveys. Thus, the counterclaim to using them is that they would require too much survey space and time to complete, and thus have to be offset with the deletion of other important quality measurements. But if everyone in the industry were to care about doctor-patient relationships, then adding 20 or 30 questions to a survey instrument, or creating a dedicated instrument that could be administered at several different time points, would not be seen as onerous.

Qualitative assessments would be invaluable to assessing features such as trust, listening, and dialogue between doctor and patient. The electronic medical record (EMR) could facilitate assessment in this regard. Using voice recording technologies that can be built into EMR software (Chavis 2015), entire exam room conversations can be recorded and then analyzed across several different encounters for the presence of various relational features in the doctor-patient interaction. Although issues around patient privacy and confidentiality might have to be addressed, the fact is a physician's own notes entered in the EMR often reflect (or should) the range of confidential issues discussed in a given encounter. Thus, the difference here is one of completeness and not whether such information should or can be collected. Once embedded in the patient's electronic health record, samples of these exam room conversations could be selected and gauged to determine the level of relational depth occurring across time, with patients from such encounters followed up with at select points to place these interactional moments with their doctor into a wider context of their general relationship with that doctor.

Sound too complex? Too expensive? That would be the standard industry response to such ideas. The technology already exists, however, and the added expense, especially for the larger health care systems and organizations employing physicians, would be the staff time required to sample conversations, listen to and assess them, administer a follow-up 10- or 15-minute survey to a small group of patients, and then disseminate the results. These added expenses might be willingly paid for by doctors or insurers if the features of relational care being assessed were, like other quality metrics, tied in meaningful ways to added incentives if performed well. In addition, to entice physicians to play along with this seemingly more intrusive form of relationship assessment, part of the overall data collection could focus on *asking them* to provide ongoing input on the degree to which they feel able to enact features like empathy and dialogue on a daily basis with their patients, and the diverse ways they attempt to provide relational care effectively within various work contexts. Such data could be quantified and tied to added incentives for select physicians who seek to innovate or overcome obstacles in their attempts to build trusting relationships with their patients.

Technology could be used in other ways to measure relational care. How about the use of a smartphone app, similar to *Yelp*, which would be available to patients for providing their doctors and health care organizations with real-time feedback on the quality of interaction with their doctors? An app like *ZocDoc* already does this for their customers, but it is far from being seen as industry standard. Every time I go to a restaurant, the existence of *Yelp!* motivates me to talk about any and all aspects of my experience soon after. Recent evidence suggests that the use of *Yelp!* to review health care providers and organizations has traction among patients (Ranard et al. 2016). There is no reason not to have something similarly available to every patient immediately after face-to-face or virtual interactions with any doctor. Even without the presence of an app, a simple e-mail survey, like the ones I receive often from third-party vendors who sell me things on Amazon, could suffice.

Ironically, this is an example of how retail thinking might be used to enhance the focus on doctor-patient relationships.

These are limited examples of how to cultivate more valid, reliable measurements of features associated with strong doctor-patient relationships. So much of the general idea is common sense when printed on the page, but would inevitably be seen as innovative and potentially transformative if adopted across the industry, particularly in the primary care sphere. There would be a necessary period of fleshing out the best ways of measuring, the right technologies to use, mechanisms for incentivizing, and the appropriate pitches to make to both doctors and patients, but it could be done. Especially if there were added dollars attached to it (e.g., *what gets paid for gets done*). Given increasing consolidation in the industry, and the embedding of doctors in large health care systems and organizations, there is reason to think that the venture capital and infrastructure required would be available.

It is important to be realistic here. In an industry wholly bought into metrics and now paying more directly for performance, it makes sense to steer the conversation toward measuring and collecting data for relational care at the same time the supporting philosophy on why such care matters is also sold. In other words, the chicken and egg must be pushed simultaneously. After all, innovations like the "patient-centered medical home" began as a few general bullets on a web site, offering little specific guidance, that captured what a few key stakeholders believed were the essential principles of good primary care. The concept only took off and gained traction once the National Committee for Quality Assurance (NCQA) conjured up an entire checklist of measurements for those principles on which providers could be assessed, compared, and incentivized.

A FEW FINAL WORDS ON THE KIND OF HEALTH CARE DELIVERY SYSTEM WE WANT

In the final sum, this book tells a troubling story about our health care delivery system and where it is headed. At its core, that story has a theme of inevitable change, particularly for doctors, patients, and their relationship with each other. There have been things lost with respect to that relationship that will never return, at least on a larger scale. How much this relationship has been damaged over the past several decades is debatable. But significant damage is done. While specialty medicine, with few exceptions, remains more about doctors as technicians rather than as relational caregivers, the field of primary care and thus medicine as a whole now suffers from an increasing dearth of relationship excellence. This is disappointing in many ways. As analyzed throughout this book, it stands to lessen the relevance of all doctors in our hearts, minds, and everyday lives. It makes us prone to believe the hype that once IBM's Watson supercomputer or some future innovation in artificial intelligence or robotics can take over the intellectual and technical aspects of their jobs, we simply will not need as many physicians. They can be automated out of existence like every other worker. It deludes us into thinking that an exam room located in a big box retail store or strip mall, staffed by shift workers, or a smartphone app that makes it easy to see some strange clinician within hours of our request are the new and improved points of contact with getting much of our primary care delivered to us. All the while, we may not much notice how things are really changing under us, and how the overall substance of our interactions with the health care delivery system is deteriorating because of our already diminished expectations and the fewer relational care experiences in our health care lives, both of which allow us to believe that what we see before us, the new normal, is the way it has to be.

In trying to articulate what relational care means to doctors and patients, and also in trying to achieve the goal of a more humane, ethical, and emotionally satisfying delivery system, critics might contend that the debate at times drifts into a sort of "rose-colored glasses" view on the past health care delivery system. By asserting that a dyadic doctor-patient relationship based on regular interpersonal contact is important, for example, we make many assumptions about the proven value of this relationship and its past glory. But here's the thing: many of those assumptions are true. We have both research and common sense supporting these. In other walks of life as well, we know how meaningful interpersonal dynamics such as trust, empathy, compassion, mutual respect, and listening are to our well-being. Successful marriages are built solidly on these features, as are religious faith, bonds between friends and family, and successful work careers.

This is not stuff made up on the fly. Certainly, the doctor-patient relationship has never consisted of a full realization of these features for all patients. Some doctors have little bedside manner. Others should never have become physicians in the first place given their lack of the empathy gene. Still others may not want deeper relationships with their patients all that much. But that particular critique does not undercut the main point being made here, which is that these relational features have been a significant part of many, many doctor-patient relationships through time, and their presence has unequivocally improved the lives of both parties to that relationship in the process, as well as helped to transform our larger society into a more caring and supportive one for its members. That is indisputable.

From having worked in and studied the health care system for several decades, I believe strongly that all of us in good measure, provider and patient alike, long for something deeply personal in health care. When we are sick, we want to be comforted and heard. We want to open up to someone we think can help us. We want to have someone we trust give us sound guidance but also the emotional support of a good friend. When we are healthy we want someone to keep us healthy, to convince us where we need to change our thinking and behavior, but also to know us well enough to respect the boundary between what we can and will not do to live healthy lives. We want a trained expert, namely a physician, to know who we are and what we have experienced, and then be ready and willing to apply that information in making decisions about what we need in health care. We also want all of this for our own family and friends.

Of course, in an ideal world no one should have to wait to see a physician as a new patient for months, or as an existing patient be unable to gain timely access to his regular doctor when he believes he needs it. We deserve better attention to the full range of details involved in our interactions with the health system, from friendlier staff to greater simplicity around things like insurance billing, making doctors' appointments, and figuring out where to go in the system. The current delivery system underperforms on so many levels that at times it boggles the mind given the money we are spending. But the marketing hype of a retail-focused health system in which a chief goal is "consumer engagement," which mostly means getting us on the hook as *buyers* likely will not solve these types of problems on more than an idiosyncratic scale, because these problems do not have easy, single-dimensional, or cheap solutions. Nor is retail thinking interested in solving them on more than a company-specific basis, given that the goal in applying this thinking is not systemwide improvement for the sake of society, doctors, patients, or the system as a whole, but rather individual company profit, market share, and growth. Innovating to solve problems such as access and convenience through a market-based system is the means to corporate growth, market share, and profit, and is not intended to provide social justice.

To conclude that strong, mutually satisfying doctor-patient relationships cannot be part of our evolving health system is to cop out for reasons that have less to do with reality and more to do with the ways in which the new and powerful corporate influences in health care see relational care between doctors and patients, that is, not as something to synergize or build upon but rather as an unwelcome rival to devoting resources to the philosophy and tactics of selling things, building brand loyalty, standardizing as much as possible, and maximizing transactional speed. Even the medical profession is complicit here. As an institution, it complains incessantly about physician shortages, yet does little to create a larger flow of doctors through its schools and residency programs, in part to protect high salaries for its in-demand workers. It creates self-fulfilling prophecies about the future role of doctors in our health system by clinging to antiquated views of its workforce and encouraging infighting. Groups of physicians cut parochial deals with industry stakeholders such as insurance companies and hospitals that make everyday life for themselves worse, in return for a few extra reimbursement dollars. Overall, the profession avoids strengthening the one aspect of its members' work that will most preserve its future cultural legitimacy, namely, relational care ability.

This story is about more than just change, though, or the inevitable evolution of an industry that must focus on many strategic imperatives at once—become less costly; keep improving quality; meet intensive access demands; and incentivize its leading organizations to earn a profit in return for advancing innovation and growth. The rhetoric of "inevitable change" may have some truth to it, but that does not mean it has to disempower both doctors and patients. It does not mean that the only viable solution is to place our trust in a market-based delivery system and the talents of large organizations. *It is complex and multifaceted, no one is denying that.* But few things in health care are truly inevitable. They are all just one or another set of policy choices and decisions, embedded within certain sociopolitical and economic contexts that push change in a specific direction based on whose interests can win out at the time. For example, we have Obamacare and then suddenly we may have something else, simply because the political party in power is different.

The essential issue when considering the doctor-patient relationship and retail thinking is about the kind of health care delivery system we want to have both in this country and elsewhere. Do we want a delivery system that is cold, impersonal, highly transactional, and focused on trying to organize itself like a well-oiled, technologically dominated assembly line? Do we want a delivery system where corporations and outside business entrepreneurs control the care rather than the individual professionals trained and socialized to have our best interests as patients at heart, even if those professionals are imperfect and some of them may be in it for other more self-interested reasons? Do we want doctors out of our lives, replaced by cool but emotionally dumb gadgets and machines? Do we want the glitz technology without the substance of human interaction?

Or do we want something different for our health care, something that retains its humanity at a level appropriate for the type of service we are receiving? After the Affordable Care Act (ACA) passed in the United States and it became clear that the system would continue to evolve as a for-profit marketplace, we were sold into thinking that the industry needed to incorporate the sorts of ideas and innovations other market-based industries use. This was a direct fault of the ACA, this casting of health care as a highly rational, numbers-driven business, full of correctible waste everywhere, and it likely will remain a fault of whatever health care laws and policies might replace it. It is also a fault of government-run health care systems like those found in Canada and Europe. On the contrary, health care is an emotional, necessarily wasteful, and highly irrational business, and that is an obvious point to anyone who has worked within it and either delivered or received care. It does not play by the normal rules of business, nor should it in many ways.

Health care services are in key ways very different from other consumer services and products we encounter in the rest of our lives. We absolutely need health care at various points in our lives, much of the time suddenly, and when we need it, we want a meaningful human feel to be present. We *choose* to buy flat-screen televisions, stop at the local Starbucks to purchase a latte, and shop for things on Amazon. We do not *need* much of what we end up having in our lives, nor do we expect these types of interactions to be deeply relational. When we check in at a Marriott or call up the Netflix service center, we expect basic politeness and perhaps the person on the other end to listen carefully and empathize with our immediate concern. We expect timely service and our basic needs addressed. But it's not like we must connect with these organizations on an extended basis so that we can feel safe enough to reveal the most personal things about ourselves that impact our health, or to confront something so profound it is life-threatening or life-changing. The hotel clerk is relational interaction at its most superficial, unimportant level, especially when we compare it to health care. Marriott and Netflix want us to believe otherwise, however, because doing so enhances their brand in our eyes, and gets us to buy more of their stuff.

Getting and keeping us healthy is not an exact science, nor will it ever be, and so doctors' work cannot have all of its "waste" work flowed out, or broken down completely into a neat little set of performance metrics or transaction steps. Yet, that is exactly what the system keeps trying to do. Building and maintaining strong relational elements like trust is not a linear process. It involves fits and starts, breakthrough moments and extended periods where no progress is apparent. Talking to each other, for example, involves lots of "waste." Trust, empathy, listening, respect—these sorts of features depend heavily on allowing for spare time and the chance for serendipity to occur in an interpersonal relationship. Much of what goes on between a doctor and patient, when it is truly working well is messy, complicated, highly idiosyncratic, and not "checklistable."

It depends more on the particular talents and experiences of the two individuals interacting with each other, on how much they know or infer about each other, than on some series of standard check boxes that read like a grocery list of staples. Those check boxes may indeed be very important for making sure the wrong limb isn't being removed or that patients in the ICU are getting the most appropriate care, or that diabetics have had their eye and foot exams at regular intervals. But they have little value for facilitating strong emotional and psychological bonds between doctor and patient. They do not help a physician know when to dig deeper with a patient or when not to do so, nor do they give patients a roadmap for how to interact with their doctor. They do not till the relational soil and ready it for planting and harvesting a wealth of interactional crops both doctor and patient use to bond, trust, and maintain a state of health together.

Is there a place for some elements of consumerist thinking, retail tactics, and market-oriented philosophies in our health care system? Absolutely. As mentioned earlier, it does not have to be an either–or question necessarily, though if it is, then give me a focus on the relational over everything else. But it makes more sense to think of it more as a question of degree and relativity. Which retail thinking and consumer-focused tactics to employ, where, and why? How does the delivery system get better at transactional excellence related to achieving goals like timelier access and convenience without undermining the ability of doctors and patients to develop strong bonds with each other? How can the health care delivery system move away from standardization toward a more variable mindset to ensure that in certain service areas where relational care is most needed it will be there? These are the sorts of questions that policy makers, industry executives, entrepreneurs and innovators, health professionals, and patients must answer. We need to have extended debate on them.

There are too many walks of our lives now where we have acquiesced our expectations for how we want to relate to others who are important to us. Too many instances where we have traded the quality of the "strong tie" interpersonal relationship for the quantity of the "weak tie" network relationship, where we have been fine with the superficial rather than the highly personal, the transactional rather than the relational. This study and all I think I know from my prior research, the research of others, and from working in health care and being a patient myself, convinces me that at least with respect to health care, we must strive to protect the human quality of one of the last industries in society that still values it, and absolutely needs it.

I end with how I began, pondering my own experiences, views, and beliefs. I worry as a patient that perhaps I will never again have a sustained relationship with a doctor of the type this book advocates. I fear I may succumb increasingly to the retail message painting me as a "health care consumer," and respond to pitches from the industry that try to sell me on the idea that I am special, that I deserve only the best in spending my health care dollar. I worry that my own expectations will continue to decline, because so much of the health care delivery experience stinks, and that I will place my trust in the big corporate organization that says it wants to take care of all of my needs so that I do not have to worry about getting around in a complicated system. I tell myself now is not the time to get complacent, or to give myself over to rhetoric and guile. Now is as good a time as any to self-reflect, self-critique, and think about how I can turn thought into action. The doctor-patient relationship cannot flourish solely through my little effort. But like anything, lots of little efforts produce bigger change. Perhaps that is how each of us should think about what we want and how to make it happen in health care.

APPENDIX

How the Study Was Conducted

This is the second full-length scholarly book in which I have used the straightforward methodological approach of talking with people and dovetailing some of what I am hearing with information gleaned from published sources to create an analysis that merits further attention by researchers, managers, policy makers, and those working in and receiving health care. As an academic who works in both a business school and school of public policy, and as someone who tries to take an applied perspective in all my work, in part because of my own experiences working in the health care industry before coming to academia, I feel compelled to examine research questions that have value for both researchers and practitioners. Thus, like my prior book (Hoff 2010), this one is a sort of hybrid treatise on a complex phenomenon, and the methodological approach reflects that hybrid character.

The research was qualitative. It was approved by the Northeastern University Institutional Review Board. I used data in the form of interviews and archival materials consisting of peer-reviewed journal articles; reports and surveys from legitimate sources such as think tanks, foundations, and professional associations; and news articles from an array of media outlets. During the time period November 2014 through February 2017 I interviewed a total of 80 primary care physicians and individuals representing the patient perspective. Forty-four of these interviews were with doctors, and the remainder with patients. My focus was on adult primary care, so my physician sample was limited to family physicians and general internists. I felt that if strong doctor-patient relationships existed, they would most likely be found within this brand of medicine. My patient sample included individuals ranging from their twenties to seventies in age. I conducted ad hoc literature reviews throughout this same time period on a variety of topics addressed in the book such as the doctor-patient relationship; consumer engagement; retail thinking and principles; health care quality; payment reform in health care; workforce issues; trends in health insurance and accreditation, performance measurement, system integration, and health care delivery; and health system innovation.

Qualitative research is inductive and idiographic. This means it is designed to capture the particular, grounded in its normal everyday context, in the hopes of illuminating more general statements regarding specific phenomena. Such an approach helps the researcher know what she or he doesn't know. Qualitative work requires neither large data sets nor adherence to statistical theory, even though some always mistakenly critique on the basis that it should involve both. Instead, it must meet a litmus test of *believability* in relation to how the data interpretations resonate for the reader (Van Maanen 1979). Using systematic methods of sampling, data collection, and data analysis (see Miles and Huberman 1994; Patton 2002; Strauss 1987) I used interview and archival data to explore the topics of interest, specifically, the doctor-patient relationship; the relational care elements associated with it such as trust, empathy, and listening; and the alignment of various retail and market-based principles with current views on and experiences with the relationship itself.

Because I was interested in something that by its traditional definition is interpersonal and dyadic, I focused my data collection in the interviews on gaining insights from two groups of individuals as parties to the relationship, obtaining descriptions of their experiences interacting with each other over time. With few exceptions the patients and doctors interviewed were not associated with each other, that is to say, the doctors were not the personal physicians of the patients. This allowed me exposure to a large number of different relationship experiences, although it limited my ability to gain perspective on the same exact relationship from two different vantage points.

I used the interviews to identify key elements of the meaning systems each of the two groups possessed regarding the doctor-patient relationship. I was interested in their views, beliefs, and sensemaking, that is, the personal and highly subjective side of their interpersonal experiences and what they learned from or thought about them. I enabled wide latitude during interviews to expound on their thoughts, trying to elicit from them real-world examples to better appreciate why they might feel or believe a certain way. In this way, I used most of each interview to listen rather than ask questions, keeping them focused on the general topics of interest but allowing what they felt was notable to emerge from our real-time conversation around their thoughts.

Doctors and patients described the "best" kinds of relational experiences with one another and provided their analysis as to why they felt they were the best. I asked them about whether or not they valued these experiences and if so how and why, trying always not to lead them in too directed a manner by naming things like trust or listening. I inserted some probes about various forms of service delivery innovation, such as the use of electronic medical records and teams to see if and how these things shaped their relational care experiences. I also tried as much as possible to get each group to "put their cards on the table" so to speak, in terms of articulating their personal beliefs regarding the worth of and possibilities for doctor-patient care that contained heavy relational elements. When contradictions or paradoxes related to their beliefs or views emerged in the conversations, which they did, I probed individuals to try and better understand what these meant for the relationship as a whole. Similar to most other interviews I have performed in the course of prior qualitative research, for many subjects, doctor and patient alike, it took no more than 10 minutes or so to get them talking candidly about their relationship experiences and views.

That said, asking people to self-reflect on something they may not think a lot about during a normal day or week, and something that may conjure up dissonant feelings of frustration, anger, or other negative emotions when they do think about it requires allowing people to pick a day and time of their choosing to talk. Above all else, I have learned from doing qualitative data collection with physicians to fit myself into their schedule, which I did. Even for patients, I was respectful of when they could be available (e.g., not during the day when working). Thus, I did interviews at all different times of the day, especially during evening hours and early morning. To facilitate flexibility in scheduling, I conducted approximately 75 percent of the interviews by phone, with the rest done in person. In addition, I spread the interviews out over a two-year period. In part, I spread the interviews out over a longer time period as part of the analytic strategy, which is detailed below.

Before beginning the book, I perused the extant literature to see if there was anything similar already available. There may have been, but my search did not yield any books of the type that I was setting out to write. I found a couple of books, for example, on how the use of computers and information technology was changing medicine (cf. Wachter 2015), but nothing specifically focused on the evolving doctor-patient relationship, told from the perspective of the participants, in the midst of an industry making a market-focused turn in delivering health care. Surprisingly, much of what is written on the doctor-patient relationship continues to take the form of opinion-editorial type laments across a range of journals, which, while helpful in identifying key big picture issues shaping the landscape, rests little on extended or systematic analysis of real data.

Information on the Interview Sample

Both the physician and patient sampling strategies were guided by a purposive, snowball sampling approach in which I sought out interviewees across a range of demographic characteristics (see Patton 2002). For physicians, my primary stratification variables of interest were age, gender, career stage (positively correlated with age), and type of employment setting (see Table A.1). The sampling strategy involved using key contacts in the primary care physician community to help introduce me to other physicians whom they knew as colleagues, even if they worked in different medical practices. Thus, there was also a convenience aspect to sample selection.

Table A.1 PHYSICIAN INTERVIEW SAMPLE

Pseudonym	Specialty	Description of Physician Participant
Maggie	Internal Medicine	Rural practice, later career
Martha	Internal Medicine	Rural practice, later career
Betsey	Internal Medicine	Rural practice, later career
Amy	Family Medicine	Urban/suburban practice, resident
Cleo	Family Medicine	Urban/suburban practice, resident
Dana	Family Medicine	Urban/suburban practice, early career
Mary	Family Medicine	Urban/suburban practice, early career
Ola	Family Medicine	Urban/suburban practice, resident
Amy	Family Medicine	Urban/suburban practice, resident
Wilma	Family Medicine	Urban/suburban practice, early career
Billy	Internal Medicine	Rural practice, later career
Bill	Family Medicine	Rural practice, later career
Ron	Family Medicine	Rural practice, later career
Steve	Internal Medicine	Rural practice, later career
Sam	Family Medicine	Rural practice, later career
Karen	Family Medicine	Urban/suburban practice, early career
Paul	Family Medicine	Urban/suburban practice, resident
Barbara	Family Medicine	Urban/suburban practice, early career
Annie	Family Medicine	Urban/suburban practice, early career
Liza	Family Medicine	Urban/suburban practice, later career
Rachel	Family Medicine	Urban/suburban practice, early career
Pete	Family Medicine	Urban/suburban practice, early career

Pseudonym	Specialty	Description of Physician Participant
Sid	Family Medicine	Urban/suburban practice, later career
Vince	Family Medicine	Urban/suburban practice, later career
Sonny	Family Medicine	Urban/suburban practice, later career
Hal	Internal Medicine	Urban/suburban practice, later career
Ronny	Family Medicine	Urban/suburban practice, later career
Bradley	Family Medicine	Urban/suburban practice, later career
Mike	Family Medicine	Urban/suburban practice, later career
Keith	Family Medicine	Urban/suburban practice, later career
Bobby	Family Medicine	Rural practice, later career
Bridget	Family Medicine	Rural practice, resident
Karl	Internal Medicine	Urban/suburban practice, later career
Burt	Internal Medicine	Urban/suburban practice, later career
Curt	Internal Medicine	Urban/suburban practice, later career
Owen	Family Medicine	Urban/suburban practice, later career
Pam	Family Medicine	Urban/suburban practice, early career
Scott	Family Medicine	Urban/suburban practice, early career
Rick	Internal Medicine	Urban/suburban practice, later career
Uma	Family Medicine	Rural practice, early career
Harry	Family Medicine	Rural practice, resident
Sarah	Family Medicine	Urban/suburban practice, resident
Olivia	Family Medicine	Urban/suburban practice, early career
Claire	Family Medicine	Urban/suburban practice, resident

There was one physician practice where I recruited 16 doctors for interviewing, with the remaining 28 interviewees spread out across 18 different medical offices.

I did not wish to talk only with older doctors who, while having more career opportunities than younger doctors to develop deep patient relationships, still had cut their relational teeth in a health care system very different from the one they work in today. I wanted them to talk about those contrasting work contexts, but I also wanted to get the perspectives of younger doctors, even residents, who had less of a past frame of reference to guide how they interpreted their current relationship experiences. Thus, I interviewed nine current primary care physician residents as part of the total group of 44 physicians. Overall, 20 physicians (including the residents) could be classified as being "early career," that is, less than 10 years of experience practicing medicine.

I wanted to survey a fairly equal number of male and female physicians, which I was able to achieve. Twenty-one of the 44 physician interviewees were female. I was particularly interested in seeing whether there were differences around the doctor-patient relationship that would emerge between male and female physicians, given the different practice styles often associated with each group. No gender-based differences emerged, however, during analysis, which surprised me a bit but also spoke to the universal nature of some of the experiences, sensemaking, and beliefs presented here, at least in terms of how most doctors perceived the best types of relationships, and how they saw various innovations, such as team care or electronic medical records. The 44 physicians worked in 19 distinct primary care practices, some of which were owned by larger corporate entities such as hospitals or health systems, and others which were group practices technically owned by the doctors but reimbursed through a variety of insurances, such as Medicare and private payers. The practices were probably equally split in terms of large-, medium-, and small-size practices (i.e., number of providers on staff). I counted any practice with fewer than five doctors as small, six to ten doctors as medium-sized, and more than ten doctors as large.

Geographically, I interviewed 12 rural and 32 urban or suburban-based doctors; with a majority of the latter group working in and around the metro Boston area. No meaningful differences were noted in the data between rural, suburban, or urban doctors. Almost all worked under the same conditions—packed daily schedules with shorter visits; patients churning in and out of their practices; a heavy emphasis on documenting and reporting quality metrics; workflows that increasingly firewalled them from more "mundane" patient care tasks (and thus more from patients); heavy use of the electronic medical record; and team care that gave responsibilities previously involving physicians over to other office personnel, such as medical assistants and nurses. A few of the practices may have had a higher percentage of more complex patients walking through the door each day, or served a more ethnically diverse population, but that was it in terms of differences.

The physician sample is representative of the larger everyday milieu in which primary care physicians now find themselves, and in that key sense getting doctors from another part of the country to talk with me would not necessarily add anything new based on the working conditions, which are similar regardless of locale. There is no empirical proof, for example, that a primary care physician working for Kaiser Permanente or Geisinger (often held up as exemplars of physician workplaces) is any less harangued, relationship driven, or relationship-capable than the next doctor, and as I said, most of my doctors worked for larger organizations with some level of "service integration." Ten of the 44 physicians were general internists (with two trained in both internal medicine and pediatrics), and the remainder were family physicians. The heavy skewing toward family medicine was not intentional, but I did probably assume that such doctors were more likely, because of their training and socialization, to place heavier emphasis on relational care with their patients. They also would be the doctors that patients would most expect to interact with them in this way.

For the 36 patients, I sought to stratify the sample based primarily on age and gender. I thought these variables would be partial proxies for other important stratifying criteria such as health status and types of care needed, which would be more difficult to obtain in advance from potential interviewees (Table A.2). The sample as a whole reflected a variety of ages and was almost equally split by gender. I did ask each patient interviewee, to the extent comfortable, to provide a snapshot of their health status at the outset of the interview, that is, whether they were in generally

Table A.2 PATIENT INTERVIEW SAMPLE

Pseudonym	Description of Patient Participant (senior is someone over 65 years of age)
Hallie	Multiple conditions/diseases, fifties
Hadley	Multiple conditions/diseases, fifties
Krystal	Healthy, fifties
Winona	Healthy, fifties
Scarlett	Healthy, twenties
Raymond	Healthy, senior male
Will	Single chronic disease, senior male
Edward	Healthy, thirties
Wanda	Healthy (past history of disease), senior female
Teddy	Healthy, thirties
Susan	Healthy, twenties

(continued)

Table A.2 CONTINUED

Pseudonym	Description of Patient Participant (senior is someone over 65 years of age)
Lucy	Healthy, twenties
Bette	Healthy, thirties
Tonya	Healthy, twenties
Wayne	Multiple conditions/diseases, senior male
Fran	Healthy (past history of disease), thirties
Darlene	Healthy, thirties
Raul	Healthy, fifties
Cliff	Healthy, fifties
Barry	Healthy (past history of disease) sixties
Bart	Multiple conditions/diseases, sixties
Janell	Healthy, forties
Jerry	Healthy, forties
Matt	Healthy, senior male
Renee	Healthy, thirties
Pete	Healthy, twenties
Rebecca	Healthy, forties
Siobhan	Healthy, fifties
Rich	Healthy, senior male
Gabrielle	Healthy, forties
Carly	Multiple conditions/diseases, thirties
Tommy	Multiple conditions/diseases, sixties
Anthony	Multiple conditions/diseases, fifties
Mia	Healthy, fifties
Grady	Multiple conditions/diseases, fifties
Donna	Healthy, forties

good health, suffered from one or more chronic diseases, had a more serious disease like cancer, or accessed the primary care system on a frequent basis. From this knowledge, I categorized eight of the interviewees as being in poorer health compared with others. These patients generally discussed accessing the health care system more than others in the sample.

Patients were recruited through personal contacts I had with several individuals, whom I interviewed for the study. These individuals introduced me to friends or family members for interviewing, although in no case did I recruit more than a couple of individuals from the same person. While pursuing the snowball sampling approach, I also took care to try and gain enough numbers of patients possessing the types of stratification features (e.g., age, gender) that interested me. There were some limitations to the patient sample. For example, almost all of the patients were white and could be considered "middle-class" in terms of how they presented such things as their employment status, insurance status, and where they lived. Only a handful of patients came from lower socioeconomic backgrounds. In theory, overall care experiences for patients from lower socioeconomic backgrounds might be different compared with white, middle-class patients, and this could affect the findings. For example, one might expect stronger relational features and deeper, longer-term doctor-patient relationships in the higher socioeconomic status (SES) group given "better insurance" and better access to doctors in their geographic locales. Or, perhaps the opposite, that is, one might think that lower SES patients, who might have more health issues, could have better ongoing relationships with a single doctor. In comparing the interview data across the two groups, however, no differences of this type emerged.

As mentioned earlier, statistical generalizability was not required for a qualitative study like this, and so a non-probability sampling scheme like that outlined here was appropriate. That said, could leaving out of the sample patients or doctors with other types of demographic characteristics bias the findings in some way? I conducted a series of comparisons in the data, for instance, between patients who were healthier versus sicker; younger versus older; male versus female; and living in urban versus suburban areas. No meaningful differences in any of the major themes or descriptions presented in the book were observed across these patient groups. They all reported similar experiences, expectations, sensemaking, and beliefs about their relationships with doctors; and what they ultimately took away from those relationships. In fact, it was striking to me how similar these types of findings were across the data set as a whole, with the physician sample also uniform across different subgroups as to the themes identified and experiences and views described.

Analyzing the Data and Arriving at Interpretations

Having conducted a lot of interview-based qualitative research over the years, I pursued a similar analytic strategy as in my prior work. Each interviewee received a pseudonym so there was no way of identifying them. All interviews, with the exception of five were digitally recorded and transcribed onto computer. I listened to each of the 75 interviews in their entirety at least once, as well as read the transcripts of all 75 interviews. For the five not recorded, I reviewed my notes taken during the interviews. Some interviews were extremely informative and so helped me to articulate preliminary findings that I sought to validate using other interviews. I also was keen on looking for specific storytelling within the interviews, and identifying participant experiences that might help to illuminate the wider themes and patterns that were emerging as I reviewed and coded across the wider data set. For example, the "low expectations" patients held of the doctor-patient relationship in primary care, described and analyzed in Chapter 5 and Chapter 6, were first identified through descriptive coding of multiple interviews, then further validated and made more specific by finding stories in select interviews that captured the essence of the descriptive finding. In this way, I went back and forth in the analytic phase between creating larger, more systematic interpretations and trying to understand anecdotes that were unique to one person's experience, yet at times held the key to better understanding what the interpretation meant at a more abstract level of analysis.

For a theme, pattern, or interpretation to emerge from the data as meaningful, it required support from a majority or more of the interviews, whether that interview sample was the entire physician and patient data set, only the physicians, or only the patients. Each interview generated approximately 20–25 double-spaced pages of text, so there was a significant amount of qualitative information to review and analyze. For a portion of the interview sample, particularly the first 20 doctor and 20 patient interviews, I used Atlas.ti software to help perform descriptive coding that could begin to isolate views, opinions, beliefs, and experiences that were similar across a portion of the given data set. I also used Atlas.ti tools like the "word find" function to isolate instances in the data where respondents were discussing things like "trust," "communication," and "respect." I did not only look for those dynamics where the actual words were explicit in the data, but instead started with textual chunks that openly talked about these words, and then examined other places in the same interview for additional discussion.

Most of the findings presented in the book have deep and widespread support within the interview sample. There are a few findings of interest, however, that may not have achieved robust support, yet were rich enough in their descriptive power to reveal some phenomenon or insight, which, although remaining somewhat exploratory or nascent, nonetheless informed questions that were of interest in the book. Thus, some findings presented in the book are there not only because of their widespread or descriptive support in the data, but also because they speak to the larger topics that piqued my interest in writing the book in the first place. They also raise questions or suggest implications that are important for thinking about the present and future viability of the doctor-patient relationship within a market-based health system.

The book is organized in the following manner: Several introductory chapters (a) describe and analyze health care delivery system forces to illuminate a contextual backdrop in which doctor-patient relationships, relational care, and our overall expectations of these phenomena are embedded; (b) highlight the importance and value of doctor-patient relationships in health care (using systematic research findings); and (c) describe and critique a core foundational philosophy of market-based, consumer-oriented health care in the modern age, namely, that of retail thinking. These first three chapters provide the grist for asking questions regarding how doctors and patients experience their interpersonal relationships, and what these experiences mean for how each group thinks about the other, in terms of expectations and preferences.

Chapters 4, 5, and 6 form the ethnographic core of the book, and the specific findings presented in each of them are analyzed in-depth at the end of the respective chapters for their implications related to management, policy, patient care, the doctor-patient relationship, and further evolution of a consumer-oriented health care system. The final chapter circles back to discuss and analyze the prospects for strong doctor-patient relationships given the experiences and beliefs of doctors and patients presented. It also offers up modest suggestions for saving relational care within a health care delivery system that is moving forward in adopting corporate care, retail thinking, service standardization, and transactional business models.

As I also noted at the end of my 2010 book, the present book is intended for a variety of audiences, and the findings and analyses offered can be construed on several levels. For instance, is the book a sustained critique on the movement of American health care delivery into a more "Walmart-like" phase of existence where patients become "consumers" and retail thinking grows ascendant? Is it about how recent external forces associated with the quality and "value" movements have undermined the more humane, relational elements of our system permanently? One could read it and go in either or both of these directions. At its core, however, the book is about the threats under which the doctor-patient relationship now exists, and how that relationship is eroding in ways that have implications for doctors, patients, and the system as a whole. If the book sounds ideological at times, that tone is justified by the substance of the interview data and analysis presented here, which suggests good reasons to be both concerned and critical.

REFERENCES

Chapter 1

Alexander, J. A., & Bae, D. (2012). Does the patient-centered medical home work? *Health Services Management Research, 25*(2), 51–59. doi:10.1001/jama.2009.691

Ashwood, J. S., Gaynor, M., Setodji, C. M., Reid, R. O., Weber, E., & Mehrotra, A. (2016). Retail clinic visits for low-acuity conditions increase utilization and spending. *Health Affairs, 35*(3), 449–455. doi: 10.1377/hlthaff.2015.0995

Baile, W. F., & Aaron, J. (2005). Patient-physician communication in oncology: past, present, and future. *Current Opinion in Oncology, 17*(4), 331–335. Retrieved from http://journals.lww.com/co-oncology/Abstract/2005/07000/Patient_physician_communication_in_oncology__past,.3.aspx

Beck, R. S., Daughtridge, R., & Sloane, P. D. (2002). Physician-patient communication in the primary care office: a systematic review. *The Journal of the American Board of Family Practice, 15*(1), 25–38. Retrieved from http://www.jabfm.org/content/15/1/25.short

Becker, E. R., & Roblin, D. W. (2008). Translating primary care practice climate into patient activation: the role of patient trust in physician. *Medical Care, 46*(8), 795–805.

Botelho, R. J. (1992). A negotiation model for the doctor-patient relationship. *Family Practice, 9*(2), 210–218. doi: 10.1097/MLR.0b013e31817919c0

Centers for Medicare and Medicaid Services. (2016a). *CAHPs.* Retrieved from https://www.cms.gov/Research-Statistics-Data-and-Systems/Research/CAHPS/

Centers for Medicare and Medicaid Services. (2016b). *MACRA*. Retrieved from https://www.cms.gov/Medicare/Quality-Initiatives-Patient-Assessment-Instruments/Value-Based-Programs/MACRA-MIPS-and-APMs/MACRA-MIPS-and-APMs.html

Challener, W. (1949). The doctor patient relationship and the right to privacy. *University of Pittsburgh Law Review, 11*(4), 624–635. Retrieved from http://heinonline.org/HOL/Page?handle=hein.journals/upitt11&div=58&g_sent=1&collection=journals#

Derksen, F., Bensing, J., & Lagro-Janssen, A. (2013). Effectiveness of empathy in general practice: a systematic review. *British Journal of General Practice, 63*(606), e76–e84. doi: https://doi.org/10.3399/bjgp13X660814

Di Blasi, Z., Harkness, E., Ernst, E., Georgiou, A., & Kleijnen, J. (2001). Influence of context effects on health outcomes: a systematic review. *The Lancet, 357*(9258), 757–762. http://dx.doi.org/10.1016/S0140-6736(00)04169-6

Estupinan, J., Kaura, A., & Fengler, K. (2014). The birth of the healthcare consumer: growing demands for choice, engagement, and experience. *StrategyAnd.* Retrieved from http://www.strategyand.pwc.com/reports/birth-of-healthcare-consumer

Fassaert, T., Van Dulmen, S., Schellevis, F., Van der Jagt, L., & Bensing, J. (2008). Raising positive expectations helps patients with minor ailments: a cross-sectional study. *BMC Family Practice, 9*(1), 1. doi: 10.1186/1471-2296-9-38

Fiscella, K., Meldrum, S., Franks, P., Shields, C. G., Duberstein, P., McDaniel, S. H., & Epstein, R. M. (2004). Patient trust: is it related to patient-centered behavior of primary care physicians? *Medical Care, 42*(11), 1049–1055. Retrieved from http://journals.lww.com/lww-medicalcare/Abstract/2004/11000/Patient_Trust__Is_It_Related_to_Patient_Centered.3.aspx

Fogarty, L. A., Curbow, B. A., Wingard, J. R., McDonnell, K., & Somerfield, M. R. (1999). Can 40 seconds of compassion reduce patient anxiety? *Journal of Clinical Oncology, 17*(1), 371–371. doi: 10.1200/JCO.1999.17.1.371

Grumbach, K., & Bodenheimer, T. (2004). Can health care teams improve primary care practice? *JAMA, 291*(10), 1246–1251. doi:10.1001/jama.291.10.1246

Hall, M. A., Dugan, E., Zheng, B., & Mishra, A. K. (2001). Trust in physicians and medical institutions: what is it, can it be measured, and does it matter? *Milbank Quarterly, 79*(4), 613–639. doi: 10.1111/1468-0009.00223

Hoff, T. (2010a). The patient-centered medical home: what we need to know more about. *Medical Care Research and Review, 67*(4), 383–392. doi: 10.1177/1077558710368550

Hoff, T. (2010b). *Practice Under Pressure: Primary Care Physicians and their Medicine in the Twenty-First Century.* New Brunswick, NJ: Rutgers University Press.

Hoff, T. (2013a). Embracing a diversified future for US primary care. *The American Journal of Managed Care, 19*(1), e9–e13. Retrieved from http://europepmc.org/abstract/med/23379778

Hoff, T. (2013b). Medical home implementation: a sensemaking taxonomy of hard and soft best practices. *Milbank Quarterly*, *91*(4), 771–810. doi: 10.1111/1468-0009.12033

Hoff, T., & Collinson, G. E. (2016). How do we talk about the physician–patient relationship? What the nonempirical literature tells us. *Medical Care Research and Review.* Advance online publication. doi: 10.1177/1077558716646685

Hoff, T., Weller, W., & DePuccio, M. (2012). The patient-centered medical home. A review of recent research. *Medical Care Research and Review, 69*(6), 619–644. doi: 10.1177/1077558712447688

Jacoby, R., Crawford, A. G., Chaudhari, P., & Goldfarb, N. I. (2011). Quality of care for two common pediatric conditions treated by convenient care providers. *American Journal of Medical Quality, 26*(1), 53–58. doi: 10.1177/1062860610375106

Kaplan, S. H., Greenfield, S., & Ware Jr, J. E. (1989). Assessing the effects of physician-patient interactions on the outcomes of chronic disease. *Medical Care, 27*(3), S110–S127. Retrieved from http://journals.lww.com/lww-medicalcare/Abstract/1989/03001/Assessing_the_Effects_of_Physician_Patient.10.aspx

Keating, N. L., Green, D. C., Kao, A. C., Gazmararian, J. A., Wu, V. Y., & Cleary, P. D. (2002). How are patients' specific ambulatory care experiences related to trust, satisfaction, and considering changing physicians? *Journal of General Internal Medicine, 17*(1), 29–39. doi: 10.1046/j.1525-1497.2002.10209.x

King, R. (1987). Technology and the doctor-patient relationship. *International Journal of Technology Assessment in Health Care, 3*(1), 11–18. https://doi.org/10.1017/S0266462300011697

Lazerow, R. (2014). Beyond the clinics: What the retail movement really means. *Advisory.* Retrieved from https://www.advisory.com/research/health-care-advisory-board/blogs/at-the-helm/2014/07/retail-medicine.

Mayer, R. C., Davis, J. H., & Schoorman, F. D. (1995). An integrative model of organizational trust. *Academy of Management Review, 20*(3), 709–734. doi: 10.5465/AMR.1995.9508080335

Mazzi, M. A., Rimondini, M., Deveugele, M., Zimmermann, C., Moretti, F., Van Vliet, L., ... Bensing, J. (2015). What do people appreciate in physicians' communication? An international study with focus groups using videotaped medical consultations. *Health Expectations, 18*(5), 1215–1226. doi: 10.1111/hex.12097

Morgan, R. M., & Hunt, S. (1999). Relationship-based competitive advantage: the role of relationship marketing in marketing strategy. *Journal of Business Research, 46*(3), 281–290. http://dx.doi.org/10.1016/S0148-2963(98)00035-6

National Institute of Diabetes and Digestive and Kidney Diseases. (2014). *The AIC Test and Diabetes.* Retrieved from https://www.niddk.nih.gov/health-information/diabetes/diagnosis-diabetes-prediabetes/a1c-test.

Ong, L. M., De Haes, J. C., Hoos, A. M., & Lammes, F. B. (1995). Doctor-patient communication: a review of the literature. *Social Science & Medicine, 40*(7), 903–918. http://dx.doi.org/10.1016/0277-9536(94)00155-M

Orth, J. E., Stiles, W. B., Scherwitz, L., Hennrikus, D., & Vallbona, C. (1987). Patient exposition and provider explanation in routine interviews and hypertensive patients' blood pressure control. *Health Psychology*, 6(1), 29. https://doi.org/10.1037/0278-6133.6.1.29

Ranard, B. L., Werner, R. M., Antanavicius, T., Schwartz, H. A., Smith, R. J., Meisel, Z. F., ... Merchant, R. M. (2016). Yelp reviews of hospital care can supplement and inform traditional surveys of the patient experience of care. *Health Affairs*, 35(4), 697–705. https://doi.org/10.1377/hlthaff.2015.1030

Schroeder, R. (2013). The seriously mentally ill older adult: perceptions of the patient–provider relationship. *Perspectives in Psychiatric Care*, 49(1), 30–40. https://doi.org/10.1111/j.1744-6163.2012.00338.x

Shorten, O. (1966). The doctor-patient relationship in surgery. *The Journal of the College of General Practitioners*, 11(1), 21–33. https://doi.org/10.1007/springerreference_61332

Simpson, M., Buckman, R., Stewart, M., Maguire, P., Lipkin, M., Novack, D., & Till, J. (1991). Doctor-patient communication: the Toronto consensus statement. *British Medical Journal*, 303(6814), 1385. https://doi.org/10.1136/bmj.303.6814.1385

Stewart, M. A. (1995). Effective physician-patient communication and health outcomes: a review. *Canadian Medical Association Journal*, 152(9), 1423.

Street, R. L., Makoul, G., Arora, N. K., & Epstein, R. M. (2009). How does communication heal? Pathways linking clinician-patient communication to health outcomes. *Patient Education and Counseling*, 74(3), 295–301. https://doi.org/10.1016/j.pec.2008.11.015

Street, R. L., & Voigt, B. (1997). Patient participation in deciding breast cancer treatment and subsequent quality of life. *Medical Decision Making*, 17(3), 298–306. https://doi.org/10.1177/0272989x9701700306

The Physicians Foundation. (2014). *2014 Survey of America's Physicians: Practice Patterns and Perspectives*. Retrieved from http://www.physiciansfoundation.org/uploads/default/2014_Physicians_Foundation_Biennial_Physician_Survey_Report.pdf:

Thom, D. H., & Campbell, B. (1997). Patient-physician trust: an exploratory study. *Journal of Family Practice*, 44(2), 169–177. Trachtenberg, F., Dugan, E., & Hall, M. A. (2005). How patients' trust relates to their involvement in medical care: trust in the medical profession is associated with greater willingness to seek care and follow recommendations. *Journal of Family Practice*, 54(4), 344–353.

Turino, G. M. (1986). The future of the doctor-patient relationship. *Bulletin of the New York Academy of Medicine*, 62(10), 1014. https://doi.org/10.1002/9781118728130.ch8

Van Berckelaer, A., DiRocco, D., Ferguson, M., Gray, P., Marcus, N., & Day, S. (2012). Building a patient-centered medical home: obtaining the patient's voice. *The Journal of the American Board of Family Medicine*, 25(2), 192–198. https://doi.org/10.3122/jabfm.2012.02.100235

Chapter 2

Agency for Healthcare Research and Quality. (2015). *2015 Chartbook: What Patients Say About Their Health Care Providers and Medical Practices.* Retrieved from https://www.cahpsdatabase.ahrq.gov/Files/2015CAHPSClinicianGroup.html

Ashwood, J. S., Gaynor, M., Setodji, C. M., Reid, R. O., Weber, E., & Mehrotra, A. (2016). Retail clinic visits for low-acuity conditions increase utilization and spending. *Health Affairs, 35*(3), 449–455. https://doi.org/10.1377/hlthaff.2015.0995

Association of American Medical Colleges. (2015). *New Physician Workforce Projections Show the Doctor Shortage Remains Significant.* Retrieved from https://www.aamc.org/newsroom/newsreleases/426166/20150303.html

Becker, S., Murphy, B., Cockrell, G., Walker, B., & Walsh, A. (2016). Private equity in healthcare: a review of 15 different niche areas. *Becker's Hospital Review.* Retrieved from http://www.beckershospitalreview.com/white-papers/private-equity-in-healthcare-a-review-of-15-niche-investment-areas.html

Campbell, S. M., McDonald, R., & Lester, H. (2008). The experience of pay for performance in English family practice: a qualitative study. *The Annals of Family Medicine, 6*(3), 228–234. https://doi.org/10.1370/afm.844

Centers for Disease Control and Prevention. (2014). Ambulatory Care Use and Physician Office Visits. Retrieved from https://www.cdc.gov/nchs/fastats/physician-visits.htm

Centers for Disease Control and Prevention. (2017). *Chronic Disease Prevention and Health Promotion: Multiple Chronic Conditions.* Retrieved from https://www.cdc.gov/chronicdisease/

Centers for Medicare and Medicaid Services. (2017). *MACRA.* Retrieved from https://www.cms.gov/Medicare/Quality-Initiatives-Patient-Assessment-Instruments/Value-Based-Programs/MACRA-MIPS-and-APMs/MACRA-MIPS-and-APMs.html

Chaudhry, B., Wang, J., Wu, S., Maglione, M., Mojica, W., Roth, E., . . . Shekelle, P. G. (2006). Systematic review: impact of health information technology on quality, efficiency, and costs of medical care. *Annals of Internal Medicine, 144*(10), 742–752. https://doi.org/10.7326/0003-4819-144-10-200605160-00125

Creswell, J. (2014). Race is on to profit from rise of urgent care. *The New York Times.* Retrieved from https://www.nytimes.com/2014/07/10/business/race-is-on-to-profit-from-rise-of-urgent-care.html?_r=2

Eijkenaar, F., Emmert, M., Scheppach, M., & Schöffski, O. (2013). Effects of pay for performance in health care: a systematic review of systematic reviews. *Health Policy, 110*(2), 115–130. https://doi.org/10.1016/j.healthpol.2013.01.008

Endeavour Partners. (2014). New White Paper: Inside Wearables (Part 2). Retrieved from https://endeavourpartners.net/inside-wearables-pt-2-new-white-paper/

Free, C., Phillips, G., Galli, L., Watson, L., Felix, L., Edwards, P., . . . Haines, A. (2013). The effectiveness of mobile-health technology-based health behaviour change or disease management interventions for health care consumers: a systematic review. *PLOS Medicine, 10*(1), e1001362. https://doi.org/10.1371/journal.pmed.1001362

Glickman, S. W., Ou, F.-S., DeLong, E. R., Roe, M. T., Lytle, B. L., Mulgund, J., . . . Schulman, K. A. (2007). Pay for performance, quality of care, and outcomes in acute myocardial infarction. *JAMA, 297*(21), 2373–2380. https://doi.org/10.2165/00151234-200705300-00029

Gold, J. (2011). Accountable Care Organizations, Explained. *National Public Radio.* Retrieved from http://www.npr.org/2011/04/01/132937232/accountable-care-organizations-explained

Health Services and Resources Administration. (2017). *Shortage Designation.* Retrieved from https://bhw.hrsa.gov/shortage-designation

Hoff, T. (2010). *Practice Under Pressure: Primary Care Physicians and their Medicine in the Twenty-First Century.* New Brunswick, NJ: Rutgers University Press.

Hoff, T. (2013). Medical home implementation: a sensemaking taxonomy of hard and soft best practices. *Milbank Quarterly, 91*(4), 771–810. https://doi.org/10.1111/1468-0009.12033

Hoff, T., & Collinson, G. E. (2016). *Provider and Team Adaptations to New Ways of Being Paid in Primary Care: Identifying Forms of Overt and Covert Adjustment.* Paper presented at the Academy Health Annual Research Meeting, Boston, MA.

Hoff, T., & DePuccio, M. (2016). Medical home implementation gaps for seniors perceptions and experiences of primary care medical practices. *Journal of Applied Gerontology,* 1–23. Advance online publication. https://doi.org/10.1177/0733464816637850

Hoff, T., & Scott, S. (2016). The strategic nature of individual change behavior: How physicians and their staff implement medical home care. *Health Care Management Review, 42*(3), 226–236. doi:10.1097/HMR.0000000000000109

Hoff, T. J., & Pohl, H. (2017). Not Your Parent's Profession: The Restratification of Medicine in the United States. Hoff, T.J., Sutcliffe, K.M, & Young, G.Y. (Eds.), *The Healthcare Professional Workforce* (pp. 23–46). New York, NY: Oxford University Press.

Hoff, T., Young, G., Collinson G. (2016). Provider and Team Adaptations to New Ways of Being Paid in Primary Care: Identifying Forms of Overt and Covert Adjustment. Poster presented at the 2016 Academy Health Meeting in Boston, MA.

Hwang, J., & Mehrotra, A. (2013). Why retail clinics failed to transform health care. *Harvard Business Review.* Retrieved from https://hbr.org/2013/12/why-retail-clinics-failed-to-transform-health-care

Institute for Healthcare Improvement. (2016). *The Triple Aim Initiative.* Retrieved from http://www.ihi.org/engage/initiatives/tripleaim/pages/default.aspx

Jackson, G. L., Powers, B. J., Chatterjee, R., Bettger, J. P., Kemper, A. R., Hasselblad, V., . . . Kendrick, A. S. (2013). The patient-centered medical home: a systematic review. *Annals of Internal Medicine, 158*(3), 169–178. https://doi.org/10.1097/hmr.0000000000000100

Jackson Healthcare. (2015). *Doctors Say Affordable Care Act Increasing Cost of Healthcare* [Press release]. Retrieved from http://www.prnewswire.com/news-releases/doctors-say-affordable-care-act-increasing-cost-of-healthcare-300104698.html

Jaspen, B. (2015). Retail clinics hit 10 million annual visits but just 2% of primary care market. *Forbes*. Retrieved from http://www.forbes.com/sites/bruce-japsen/2015/04/23/retail-clinics-hit-10-million-annual-visits-but-just-2-of-primary-care-market/#7425ea303891

Kutscher, B. (2015). Why private-equity firms are buying up primary-care practices. *Modern Healthcare*. Retrieved from http://www.modernhealthcare.com/article/20150418/MAGAZINE/304189980

Lehman, S. (2015). Fitness apps lack evidence-based tools. *Reuters Health*. Retrieved from http://www.reuters.com/article/us-apps-fitness-behavior-idUSKBN0KT2GU20150120

Merritt Hawkins. (2014). *Physician Appointment Wait Times and Medicaid and Medicare Acceptance Rates*. Retrieved from https://www.merritthawkins.com/uploadedfiles/merritthawkings/surveys/mha2014waitsurvpdf.pdf

Muhlestein, D. (2015). Growth and dispersion of accountable care organizations in 2015. *Health Affairs*. Retrieved from http://healthaffairs.org/blog/2015/03/31/growth-and-dispersion-of-accountable-care-organizations-in-2015-2/

National Business Coalition on Health. (2017). *Value Based Purchasing: A Definition*. Retrieved from http://www.nationalalliancehealth.org/Value-based-Purchasing-A-Definition

National Committee for Quality Assurance. (2016). *HEDIS & Performance Measurement*. Retrieved from http://www.ncqa.org/hedis-quality-measurement

Nielsen, M., Gibson, A., Buelt, L., Grundy, P., & Grumback, K. (2016). The patient-centered medical home's impact on cost and quality. *Annual Review of Evidence, 2014–2015*. Retrieved from https://www.pcpcc.org/resource/patient-centered-medical-homes-impact-cost-and-quality-2014-2015

Powell, W. W., & DiMaggio, P. J. (2012). *The New Institutionalism in Organizational Analysis*. Chicago, IL: University of Chicago Press.

Robbins, K. (2016). Healthcare Marketing Responds to Tectonic Shift in Consumer Behavior. *ResponseMine*. Retrieved from http://www.responsemine.com/healthcare-marketing-responds-consumer-behavior/

Rosenthal, E. (2014). Apprehensive, many doctors shift to jobs with salaries. *The New York Times*. Retrieved from http://healthymaryland.org/wp-content/uploads/2012/11/Apprehensive-Many-Doctors-Shift-to-Jobs-With-Salaries.pdf

Rosenthal, M. B., & Dudley, R. A. (2007). Pay-for-performance: will the latest payment trend improve care? *JAMA, 297*(7), 740–744. doi: 10.1001/jama.297.7.740

Rosenthal, M. B., & Frank, R. G. (2006). What is the empirical basis for paying for quality in health care? *Medical Care Research and Review, 63*(2), 135–157. https://doi.org/10.1177/1077558705285291

Ryan, J., Doty, M., Hamel, L., Norton, M., Abrams, M., & Brodie, A. (2015). *Primary Care Providers' Views of Recent Trends in Health Care Delivery and Payment.* Washington, DC: The Commonwealth Fund and The Kaiser Family Foundation.

Ryan, R. M., & Deci, E. L. (2000). Self-determination theory and the facilitation of intrinsic motivation, social development, and well-being. *American Psychologist, 55*(1), 68–79. https://doi.org/10.1037//0003-066x.55.1.68

Singleton, T., & Miller, P. (2015). The physician employment trend: what you need to know. *Family Practice Management, 22*(4), 11.

Starr, P. (1982). *The Social Transformation of American Medicine: The Rise of a Sovereign Profession and the Making of a Vast Industry.* New York, NY: Basic Books.

The Physicians Foundation. (2008). *The Physicians' Perspective: Medical Practice in 2008.* Retrieved from http://www.physiciansfoundation.org/uploads/default/PF_Medical_Practice_Report_2008.pdf

The Physicians Foundation. (2014). *2014 Survey of America's Physicians: Practice Patterns and Perspectives.* Retrieved from http://www.physiciansfoundation.org/uploads/default/2014_Physicians_Foundation_Biennial_Physician_Survey_Report.pdf:

U.S. Department of Health and Human Services. (2016). *20 million people have gained health insurance coverage because of the Affordable Care Act, new estimates show* [Press release]. Retrieved from https://www.hhs.gov/about/news/2016/03/03/20-million-people-have-gained-health-insurance-coverage-because-affordable-care-act-new-estimates

Urgent Care Association of America. (2017). *Industry FAQs.* Retrieved from http://www.ucaoa.org/?page=IndustryFAQs#Primary%20Care

Wachter, R. M. (2016). How measurement fails doctors and teachers. *The New York Times.* Retrieved from https://www.nytimes.com/2016/01/17/opinion/sunday/how-measurement-fails-doctors-and-teachers.html

Werner, R. M., Duggan, M., Duey, K., Zhu, J., & Stuart, E. A. (2013). The patient-centered medical home: an evaluation of a single private payer demonstration in New Jersey. *Medical Care, 51*(6), 487–493. https://doi.org/10.1097/mlr.0b013e31828d4d29

West, D. R., Radcliff, T. A., Brown, T., Cote, M. J., Smith, P. C., & Dickinson, W. P. (2012). Costs associated with data collection and reporting for diabetes quality improvement in primary care practices: a report from SNOCAP-USA. *The Journal of the American Board of Family Medicine, 25*(3), 275–282. https://doi.org/10.3122/jabfm.2012.03.110049

Chapter 3

Agency for Healthcare Research and Quality. (2014). *2014 Chartbook: What Patients Say About Their Health Care Providers and Medical Practices*. Retrieved from https://www.cahpsdatabase.ahrq.gov/files/2014CAHPSClinicianGroup.htm

Booz & Co. (2008). Health care's retail solution: a consumer-focused cure for the industry. *Strategy+Business*. Retrieved from http://www.strategyand.pwc.com/media/file/Health_Cares_Retail_Solution.pdf

Borchardt, D. (2017). Macy's store closures could cause billions of dollars in loan losses. *Forbes*. Retrieved from http://www.forbes.com/sites/debraborchardt/2017/01/05/macys-store-closures-could-cause-billions-of-dollars-in-loan-losses/#75120120460d

Bureau of Labor Statistics. (2017). *Occupational Outlook Handbook: Medical Assistants*. Retrieved from https://www.bls.gov/ooh/healthcare/medical-assistants.htm

Harding, E. (2013). Personal details in smartphone fitness apps 'sold to other firms': 20 most used products pass information to nearly 70 companies. *Daily Mail*. Retrieved from http://www.dailymail.co.uk/news/article-2409486/Personal-details-smartphone-fitness-apps-sold-firms-20-used-products-pass-information-nearly-70-companies.html

Hoff, T. (2013). Embracing a diversified future for US primary care. *The American Journal of Managed Care, 19*(1), e9–e13.

Kelly, D. L. (2011). *Applying Quality Management in Healthcare: A Systems Approach*. Washington, DC: Health Administration Press.

National Retail Federation. (2015). *Top 100 Retailers Chart 2015*. Retrieved from https://nrf.com/2015/top100-table

Punke, H. (2015). Number of 5-star hospitals decreases dramatically in CMS Hospital Compare update. *Becker's Hospital Review*. Retrieved from http://www.beckershospitalreview.com/quality/number-of-5-star-hospitals-decreases-dramatically-in-cms-hospital-compare-update.html

Scheffler, R. M., Arnold, D. R., Fulton, B. D., & Glied, S. A. (2016). Differing impacts of market concentration on Affordable Care Act marketplace premiums. *Health Affairs, 35*(5), 880–888. https://doi.org/10.1377/hlthaff.2015.1229

Smith, W. R. (1956). Product differentiation and market segmentation as alternative marketing strategies. *The Journal of Marketing, 21*(1) 3–8. https://doi.org/10.2307/1247695

Temkin Ratings. (2017). Retrieved from http://temkinratings.com/

Untouchable Intangibles. (2014). *The Economist*. Retrieved from http://www.economist.com/news/business/21614153-sometimes-you-see-brands-balance-sheet-sometimes-you-dont-untouchable-intangibles

Welfare, A. (2017). The five principles of retail. *Marketing Donut.* Retrieved from http://www.marketingdonut.co.uk/marketing-strategy/retail/the-five-principles-of-retail

Wikipedia. (2017). *Retail.* Retrieved from https://en.wikipedia.org/wiki/Retail

Chapter 4

Granovetter, M. S. (1973). The strength of weak ties. *American Journal of Sociology, 78*(6), 1360–1380. https://doi.org/10.1016/b978-0-12-442450-0.50025-0

Larson, M. S. (1977). The Rise of Professionalism: A Sociological Analysis. Oakland: University of California Press.

Mayer, R. C., Davis, J. H., & Schoorman, F. D. (1995). An integrative model of organizational trust. *Academy of Management Review, 20*(3), 709–734. doi: 10.5465/AMR.1995.9508080335

Ryan, J., Doty, M., Hamel, L., Norton, M., Abrams, M., & Brodie, A. (2015). *Primary Care Providers' Views of Recent Trends in Health Care Delivery and Payment.* Washington, DC: The Commonwealth Fund and The Kaiser Family Foundation.

Shanafelt, T. D., Dyrbye, L. N., Sinsky, C., Hasan, O., Satele, D., Sloan, J., & West, C. P. (2016). Relationship between clerical burden and characteristics of the electronic environment with physician burnout and professional satisfaction. *Mayo Clinic Proceedings, 91*(7), 836–848. https://doi.org/10.1016/j.mayocp.2016.05.007

Spangler, E. (1986). *Lawyers for Hire: Salaried Professionals at Work.* New Haven CT: Yale University Press.

Starr, P. (1982). *The Social Transformation of American Medicine: The Rise of a Sovereign Profession and the Making of a Vast Industry.* New York, NY: Basic Books.

The Physicians Foundation. (2014). *2014 Survey of America's Physicians: Practice Patterns and Perspectives.* Retrieved from http://www.physiciansfoundation.org/uploads/default/2014_Physicians_Foundation_Biennial_Physician_Survey_Report.pdf

Chapter 6

Ashwood, J. S., Gaynor, M., Setodji, C. M., Reid, R. O., Weber, E., & Mehrotra, A. (2016). Retail clinic visits for low-acuity conditions increase utilization and spending. *Health Affairs, 35*(3), 449–455. https://doi.org/10.1377/hlthaff.2015.0995

Beck, M. (2016). Can a death-predicting algorithm improve care? *The Wall Street Journal.* Retrieved from http://www.wsj.com/articles/can-a-death-predicting-algorithm-improve-care-1480702261

Booz & Co. (2008). Health care's retail solution: a consumer-focused cure for the industry. *Strategy+Business.* Retrieved from http://www.strategyand.pwc.com/media/file/Health_Cares_Retail_Solution.pdf

Centers for Medicare and Medicaid Services. (2016). *MACRA.* Retrieved from https://www.cms.gov/Medicare/Quality-Initiatives-Patient-Assessment-Instruments/Value-Based-Programs/MACRA-MIPS-and-APMs/MACRA-MIPS-and-APMs.html

Flaherty, T. B., Dahlstrom, R., & Skinner, S. J. (1999). Organizational values and role stress as determinants of customer-oriented selling performance. *Journal of Personal Selling & Sales Management, 19*(2), 1–18. Retrieved from http://www.jstor.org/stable/40471718

House, R. J., & Rizzo, J. R. (1972). Role conflict and ambiguity as critical variables in a model of organizational behavior. *Organizational Behavior and Human Performance, 7*(3), 467–505. https://doi.org/10.1016/0030-5073(72)90030-x

IBM. (2016). *Siemens Healthineers and IBM Watson Health Forge Global Alliance for Population Health Management* [Press release]. Retrieved from http://www-03.ibm.com/press/us/en/pressrelease/50760.wss

IBM. (2017). *IBM Care Management.* Retrieved from https://www-01.ibm.com/software/city-operations/smartercare/solutions/

Institute of Medicine. (2001). *Crossing the Quality Chasm: A New Health System for the 21st Century.* Washington, DC: National Academies Press.

Piko, B. F. (2006). Burnout, role conflict, job satisfaction and psychosocial health among Hungarian health care staff: a questionnaire survey. *International Journal of Nursing Studies, 43*(3), 311–318. https://doi.org/10.1016/j.ijnurstu.2005.05.003

Ryan, R. M., & Deci, E. L. (2000). Self-determination theory and the facilitation of intrinsic motivation, social development, and well-being. *American Psychologist, 55*(1), 68. https://doi.org/10.1037//0003-066x.55.1.68

Shanafelt, T. D., Hasan, O., Dyrbye, L. N., Sinsky, C., Satele, D., Sloan, J., & West, C. P. (2015). Changes in burnout and satisfaction with work-life balance in physicians and the general US working population between 2011 and 2014. *Mayo Clinic Proceedings, 90*(12), 1600–1613. https://doi.org/10.1016/j.mayocp.2015.08.023

The Beryl Institute. (2017). *State of Patient Experience Benchmarking.* Retrieved from http://www.theberylinstitute.org/?page=PXBENCHMARKING

The Physicians Foundation. (2014). *2014 Survey of America's Physicians: Practice Patterns and Perspectives.* Retrieved from http://www.physiciansfoundation.org/uploads/default/2014_Physicians_Foundation_Biennial_Physician_Survey_Report.pdf:

Volpp, K. G., Asch, D. A., Galvin, R., & Loewenstein, G. (2011). Redesigning employee health incentives—lessons from behavioral economics. *New England Journal of Medicine, 365*(5), 388–390. https://doi.org/10.1056/nejmp1105966

Chapter 7

Abbott, A. (1988). *The System of Professions: An Essay on the Division of Labor.* Chicago, IL: The University of Chicago Press.

Association of American Medical Colleges. (2016). *Workforce Data and Reports.* Retrieved from https://www.aamc.org/data/workforce/reports

Bryant, M. (2016). What's Up with Apple in Healthcare? *Healthcaredive.* Retrieved from http://www.healthcaredive.com/news/whats-up-with-apple-in-healthcare/429706/

Caryn, R.R. (2014). 15-Minute Visits Take A Toll On The Doctor-Patient Relationship. *KHN.* Retrieved from http://khn.org/news/15-minute-doctor-visits/

Chavis, S. (2015). Marrying voice and text within the EHR. *For The Record, 27*(4), 22. Retrieved from http://www.fortherecordmag.com/archives/0415p22.shtml

Collective Bargaining for Employed Physicians. (2016). *AAFP.* Retrieved from http://www.aafp.org/practice-management/payment/collective-bargaining.html

Deloitte Center for Health Solutions. (2012). *The U.S. Healthcare Market: A Strategic View of Consumer Segmentation.* Retrieved from https://www2.deloitte.com/content/dam/Deloitte/us/Documents/life-sciences-health-care/us-lshc-health-care-market-consumer-segmentation.pdf

Dow, A., & Reeves, S. (2016). *How Health Professional Training Will and Should Change The Healthcare Professional Workforce.* New York, NY: Oxford University Press.

Hoff, T. (2010). *Practice Under Pressure: Primary Care Physicians and their Medicine in the Twenty-First Century.* New Brunswick, NJ: Rutgers University Press.

Hoff, T. J. (2001). The physician as worker: what it means and why now? *Health Care Management Review, 26*(4), 53–70. https://doi.org/10.1097/00004010-200110000-00006

Hoff, T. J., & Pohl, H. (2016). Not Your Parent's Profession: The Restratification of Medicine in the United States. Hoff, T.J., Sutcliffe, K.M, & Young, G.Y. (Eds.), *The Healthcare Professional Workforce* (pp. 23–46). New York, NY: Oxford University Press.

IBM. (2016). *IBM Watson Health: Welcome to the Cognitive Era of Health.* Retrieved from https://www.ibm.com/watson/health/

Kaiser Family Foundation and Health Research Educational Trust. (2016) Employer Health Benefits Survey. Retrieved from http://kff.org/health-costs/report/2016-employer-health-benefits-survey/.

Langewitz, W., Denz, M., Keller, A., Kiss, A., Rütimann, S., & Wössmer, B. (2002). Spontaneous talking time at start of consultation in outpatient clinic: cohort study. *BMJ, 325*(7366), 682–683. https://doi.org/10.1136/bmj.325.7366.682

Leffell, D. J. (2013). The doctor's office as union shop. *The Wall Street Journal.* Retrieved from http://www.wsj.com/articles/SB10001424127887323375204578270401138739978

Massachusetts General Hospital. (2017). *Concierge Medicine*. Retrieved from https://www.massgeneral.org/appointments/forms/concierge-medicine.aspx

Mercer, S. W., Maxwell, M., Heaney, D., & Watt, G. C. (2004). The consultation and relational empathy (CARE) measure: development and preliminary validation and reliability of an empathy-based consultation process measure. *Family Practice, 21*(6), 699–705. https://doi.org/10.1093/fampra/cmh621

Mercer. (2016) *Mercer Survey: Health Benefit Cost Growth Slows to 2.4% in 2016 as Enrollment in High Deductible Plans Climbs* [Press release]. Retrieved from https://www.mercer.com/newsroom/national-survey-of-employer-sponsored-health-plans-2016.html

Neumann, M., Edelhäuser, F., Tauschel, D., Fischer, M. R., Wirtz, M., Woopen, C., . . . Scheffer, C. (2011). Empathy decline and its reasons: a systematic review of studies with medical students and residents. *Academic Medicine, 86*(8), 996–1009. https://doi.org/10.1097/acm.0b013e318221e615

Page, L. (2016). Would unions really help doctors get what they want? *Medscape.* http://www.medscape.com/viewarticle/866869

Pearson, S. D., & Raeke, L. H. (2000). Patients' trust in physicians: many theories, few measures, and little data. *Journal of General Internal Medicine, 15*(7), 509–513. https://doi.org/10.1046/j.1525-1497.2000.11002.x

Rabin, R. (2014). 15-minute visits take a toll on the doctor-patient relationship. *Kaiser Health News.* Retrieved from http://khn.org/news/15-minute-doctor-visits/

Ranard, B. L., Werner, R. M., Antanavicius, T., Schwartz, H. A., Smith, R. J., Meisel, Z. F., . . . Merchant, R. M. (2016). Yelp reviews of hospital care can supplement and inform traditional surveys of the patient experience of care. *Health Affairs, 35*(4), 697–705. https://doi.org/10.1377/hlthaff.2015.1030

Riess, H., Kelley, J. M., Bailey, R. W., Dunn, E. J., & Phillips, M. (2012). Empathy training for resident physicians: a randomized controlled trial of a neuroscience-informed curriculum. *Journal of General Internal Medicine, 27*(10), 1280–1286. https://doi.org/10.1007/s11606-012-2063-z

Scheiber, N. (2016). Doctors unionize to resist the medical machine. *The New York Times.* Retrieved from http://www.nytimes.com/2016/01/10/business/doctors-unionize-to-resist-the-medical-machine.html?_r=2

Schwartzein, R. M. (2015). Getting the right medical students: nature versus nurture. *The New England Journal of Medicine, 372*(17), 1586–1587. https://doi.org/10.1056/nejmp1501440

Starr, P. (1982). *The Social Transformation of American Medicine: The Rise of a Sovereign Profession and the Making of a Vast Industry.* New York, NY: Basic Books.

Thom, D. H., Hall, M. A., & Pawlson, L. G. (2004). Measuring patients' trust in physicians when assessing quality of care. *Health Affairs, 23*(4), 124–132. https://doi.org/10.1377/hlthaff.23.4.124

Triggle, N. (2016). Junior doctors' strike: Second all-out stoppage hits NHS. *BBC.* Retrieved from http://www.bbc.com/news/health-36145686

REFERENCES

UAPD. (2016). *All Doctors Need a Union—A Union like UAPD*. Retrieved from https://www.uapd.com/all-doctors-need-a-union/

Appendix

Hoff, T. (2010). *Practice Under Pressure: Primary Care Physicians and their Medicine in the Twenty-First Century*. New Brunswick, NJ: Rutgers University Press.

Miles, M.B. & Huberman, A.M. (1994). *Qualitative Data Analysis: An Expanded Sourcebook*. Thousand Oaks, CA: Sage Publications.

Patton, M.Q. (2002). *Qualitative Research and Evaluation Methods*. Thousand Oaks, CA: Sage Publications.

Strauss, A. (1987). *Qualitative Analysis for Social Scientists*. New York, NY: Cambridge University Press.

Van Maanen, J. (1979). Reclaiming qualitative methods for organizational research: a preface. *Administrative Science Quarterly, 24*(4), 520–526. doi:10.2307/2392358

Wachter, R. (2015). *The Digital Doctor: Hope, Hype, and Harm at the Dawn of Medicine's Computer Age*. New York, NY: McGraw-Hill Books.

ABOUT THE AUTHOR

Timothy J. Hoff, PhD, is Professor of Management, Healthcare Systems, and Health Policy at Northeastern University and Visiting Associate Fellow at Oxford University. He has worked in and studied the U.S. health care system for three decades. His research has won national awards from major professional academic societies, and Dr. Hoff is a nationally recognized expert on physician behavior, health care reform and innovation, primary care system transformation, and health workforce issues.

INDEX

References to tables are indicated with an italicized *t*.